# Healing Postures
# Of
# the 18 Siddhas

*By*

*Rudra Shivananda*

*Alight Publications*

*2007*

# Healing Postures of the 18 Siddhas

By Rudra Shivananda

First Edition Published in November 2007

Alight Publications
PO Box 930
Union City, CA 94587

*http://www.Alightbooks.com*

ISBN 1-931833-28-1

Printed in the United States of America

Dedicated

to the

# Immortal Siddhas

That Guide and Inspire

All of Us

# Healing Postures of the 18 Siddhas

## Contents

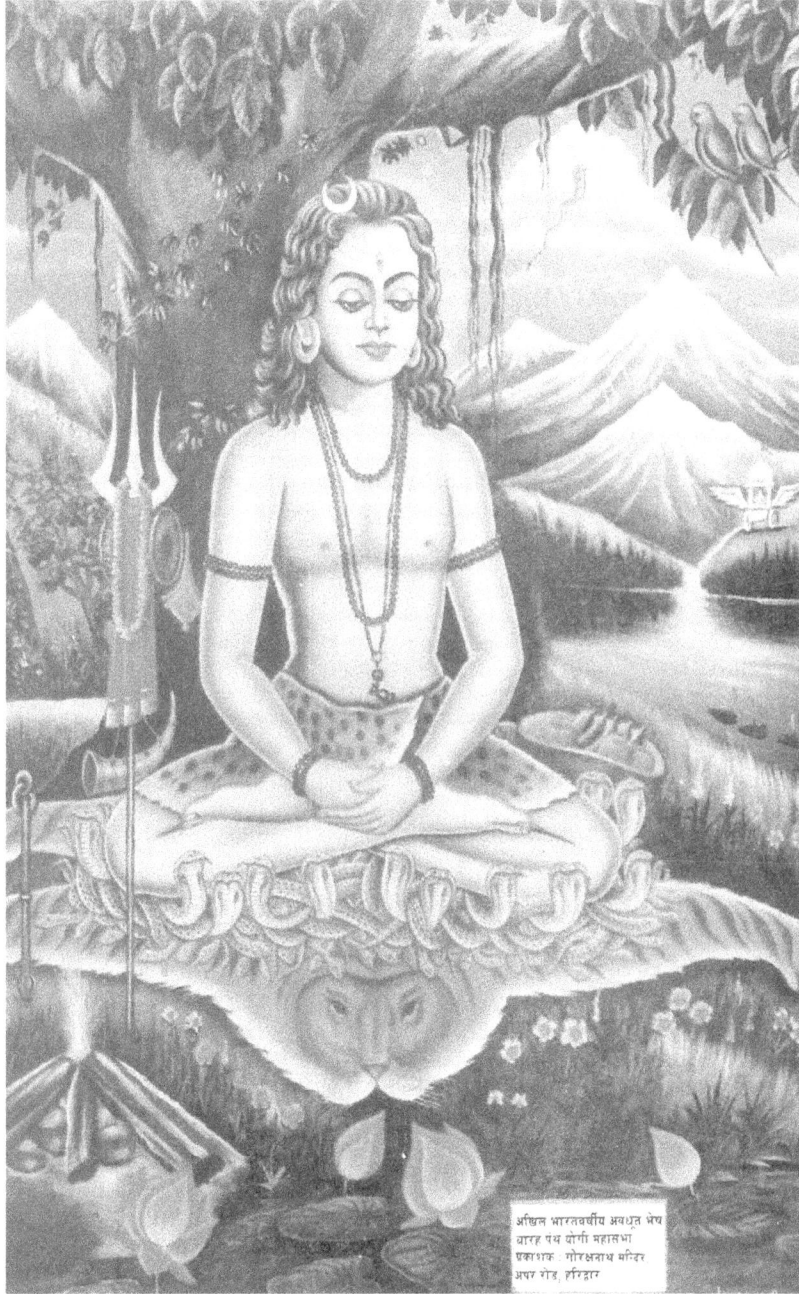

अखिल भारतवर्षीय अवधूत भेष
बारह पंथ योगी महासभा
एकाडक : गोरक्षनाथ मन्दिर
अपर रोड, हरिद्वार

Shiva-Gorakasha-Babaji

*In the beginning, we aspire to the Divine with*
*"That (Divine) I am"*
*while in the ultimate, we realise,*
*"I am That (Divine)"*

# Introduction

Yoga is not the popular physical exercise routines that have become popular among the health conscious. It is not the breathing techniques that release stress and improve energy level. It is not the meditation techniques that help one to control the mind and understand reality. Yoga is all of the above and more. Yoga is a vast and deep human enterprise formulated by sages long lost in the mist of time to enable the experience of reality and the spiritual evolution that is the unrealized human birthright. Yoga is the continuum of bliss that accompany various levels of superconscious states that are experienced during the process of Self-Realization. Yoga is true and everlasting happiness.

The postures or asanas given in the present series are a few of the hundreds of postures that can be practised by those who specialize in this area. They have been chosen because of their considerable physical, energetic and mental benefits. They have been approved and taught by the Masters of Yoga for many centuries as a preliminary to the more advanced yoga practices that usually require initiation and personal guidance. Taming the body is a pre-requisite for higher intiations into controlling energy flow and controlling the thoughts and emotions that prevent us from being happy.

Even these postures have deep effects in our psycho-energetic body-mind complex when performed with awareness. They help to develop flexiblity and strength as well as a steadiness of the body which is essential for meditation. It is not necessary to perform them like Olympic gymnastics with points taken away for an arm which is off the optimum degree or the legs not a "perfect 10" straight. Each of us have our limitations and strengths and we can train ouselves to improve and stretch ourselves a little more over time.

The purpose of this book is to introduce a very effective Yoga Posture Series. **It is not meant for those who have never practised postures before**. Those who have some experience with asanas can best benefit from it. In the modern Yoga Studio, the students are led by their instructor and they also like the group atmosphere. Learning to do the postures by yourself and from a book is a different, although equally satisfying exercise.

This series of 18 postures have been popular in India for many generations -- there are many variations of them taught in many parts of the India. This particular set was learnt by a South Indian called Yogi Ramaiah who brought it to USA in the 1970s and incorporated it into the sacred science of Self-Realization called Kriya Yoga. In the 1990s, one of his students M. Govindan has continued the work of disseminating this practice throughout the world.

**My contribution in presenting the series has been to provide two additional crucial elements to the postures which has been left out in previous efforts of dissemination. These two elements serve to elevate the postures into higher dimensions of yogic practice.** It was a necessary part of early efforts of presenting Yoga to the West, that a lot of simplifications were needed for the unprepared students to benefit from the practices.

The first element that has been added back is **the use of affirmations** -- these are presented here primarily in English. Affirmations are powerful means of de-programming and re-programming our psyche so as to eliminate emotional and mental toxins. Their use duirng the postures are especially effective because of the focus and awareness that is brought to bear during the holding phase - the mind is very susceptible to the affirmations. They have been chosen carefully to correspond to particular postures which affect certain parts of the physical and energetic bodies. Please note that in Yoga it is common to assume a model of our being which comprises of the physical body with a series of subtler bodies, much like the layering of clothing that we are familiar with. A common 5-Body model will comprise of the physical, energetic, emotional, mental and spiritual bodies. The soul wears these bodies just like your physical body wear clothing. Each posture affects not only the physical body but the energetic and emotional bodies which in turn has some affect on the mental body. The affirmations have a stronger effect on the emotional and mental bodies and therefore serve to complete the work of the posture.

The second element that has been added back is the connection with **a spiritual focus** which is represented by the name of a particular Master of Yoga, also called a Siddha or Perfected One. This might seem rather mysterious and irrevelant to those who only wish to take the physcial benefits of the postures. However, for the spiritual benefits, a connection with this higher dimension is necessary.

2

At first sight, this might seem far removed from the practice of Yoga postures one is used to seeing in the popular periodicals. It is the next level of high performance to connect with the specific energies and consciousness that are embodied by the particular Master of Yoga. For instance, the practice of the 7th posture attunes one to the energy of Bhoganath who embodies the consciousness of scientific discovery among other things - this completes the circle from physical to consciousness. Can one perform the asanas without knowing about this dimension? Yes, but when one becomes aware of the added dimension, the experience of the posture is enchanced.

The Masters who are associated with these postures are collectively called the 18 Siddhas - there are 18 of them who are part of the very fabric of the Yogic Tradition. Why eighteen and not more? There is a tradition of the Nine Naths, the primordial Lords of Creation, the greatest of "yogis," and from this has manifested the 18 Siddhas, who can be resolved back to the Nine. Alternatively, there are 18 Siddhis or special powers such as becoming as large as the largest star or as small as the smallest atomic particle, and those who have all these powers are called the 18 Siddhas.

A brief note about each of the 18 Siddhas has been given before the asanas to help the practitioner get a feel for the associated consciousness.

There are even more elements of experience which can be added to the posture practice such as the breathing patterns and muscular locks or gestures, but they require very specific guidance and cannot be safely given in a book. In general, inhalation and exhalation will follow the proper movement of the asanas and there need not be any concern with it at this stage.

There are many benefits from each posture and some of them has been listed. Under certain conditions, it is not advisable to practice certain postures. For instance, those with high blood pressure or slipped cervical disc should avoid posture #3, the shoulder stand. Common sense and knowledge of your own body are the most important factors for the successful and painless practice of the Posture series.

I've also included a note on diet as well as detailed guidelines for the practice - please do read them. A yogic practitioner is an experimenter who is open to new situations and recommendations, keeping those that work and discarding those that do not. **Develop the yogic attitude and open yourself to the higher dimensions of Posture practice. Develop the habit of practising breathing techniques and meditation after the asanas.** A simple but effective set is given as well. Practice and experiment.

# A Proper Diet

There is no such thing as a diet than is suitable for everyone. In the yogic tradition, people are categorized into three major groups called doshas or physical constitutions and there are different food suitable for the different doshas. Books have been written on such subjects and we need not try to cover them superficially - you are invited to do some research yourself.

The keys to a proper diet are:

1. Eat food that is fresh - the longer a food has been lying around or stored such as in tins, the less vitality it retains and therefore you would need to eat more bulk just to obtain the requisite energy. The fresher the food the more vital.

2. Eat food that is in season -- fruits and vegetables which are out of season will need to be forced by artificial means to be available or shipped long distances. Either way, such food will not be sufficiently nutritious.

3. Avoid highly processed food -- processing eliminates critical nutrients from the food.

4. Eat a balanced diet -- grains, fruit, nuts, vegetable and protein sources. Add roughage which is needed for proper elimination and colon health. Add herbal, vitamin, and mineral supplements because there is a deficit of them in the normal food grown in the over-farmed soil of many countries.

5. Eliminate red-meat if possible as there are a lot of toxins which are associated with meat and red-meat especially. It is not necessary to be a vegetarian to practice Yoga, but it can be helpful to lessen the load of the body. A gradual dietary improvement can be made by eating more fish and less of other meats.

# Guidelines for the 18 Postures

1.  It is good to warm-up by walking in place with swinging arms for a minute or two; rotating the shoulders; moving the head up and down and rotating it clockwise. This is especially beneficial when you've just gotten up in the morning.

2.  The postures should be performed in stages. One should perform them according to one's present state of flexibility and strength such that one can stop without strain or fear of pain.

3.  Sequence: The postures are given in an order to ensure their complementary nature, ie, they are in pairs, and should be so practiced. If you practice posture number 9, then you should do posture number 10 to complement it.

4.  Breathing should be even and smooth. Exhalation can be used to release tension and stress in tight muscles or tendons. Breathing should always be through the nose.

4.  The postures should be done with awareness. This is necessary to integrate and harmonize the 5 levels of our being - physical, energetic, emotional, mental, and spiritual. What effects the physical body will have profound effects on the other levels of our being. It is necessary to be conscious of the movements of the postures, sensations of the body, movement of the life-force energy or *prana* and concentration on the appropriate energy center or *chakra*. It is also important to be aware of the thoughts and emotions that arise during the various phases of the posture and there should be a non-judgemental attitude - one of acceptance. Awareness is the key to differentiate between an exercise routine and a yoga posture.

5.  After finishing each posture, relax for at least 30 seconds. **This is a key feature and should not be neglected, as the healing benefits are realized during the rest periods**.

6.  Most of the postures have a holding or static phase and a moving or dynamic phase. The dynamic phase is meant to increase flexibility, improve blood circulation, loosen the muscles and joints, as well as releasing energy blocks. The static phase have more subtle and powerful effects on the energy and mental bodies. They are meant to message the internal organs and to strengthen the nervous system. The static phase also brings about a tranquility of the mind and prepares the body-mind complex for meditation.

7. Practice detachment. Letting go of emotions and thoughts which arise during the postures is another key differentiator between the healing postures and physical exercises. Emotional traumas are stored in the muscles and fascia of the physical body and cause stiffness and pain to occur over time. By pressing on different parts of the body during the postures, the traumas are released and you may experience a variety of pleasant or unpleasant replays of past emotions. It is best to let go of them rather than dwelling on them.

8. There are therapeutic benefits to the postures which can experienced best with consistent daily practice. **The postures are not meant to replace medical treatment but only to supplement them.**

9. The place of practice should be well ventilated, clean and without obstructions. It is usually best to perform the postures early in the morning before breakfast or in the evening before dinner. The postures should not be done immediately after a meal -- there should be at least a two hour interval.

10. Wear comfortable clothing that are not tight or restrictive. Remove all jewellery and wristwatches that can cause discomfort during the practice.

11. Props: folded blanket to ease discomfort to any part of the body -- it is especially useful for the neck area during the shoulder stand, topsy-turvy and plough poses. A wall can also provide support for the legs during those poses.

12. It is recommended that proper hygiene be taken, such as bathing before the postures -- this helps to relax the body as well as open up the skin, removing toxins. One should not be working up a sweat during this posture series and so it is not necessary to bath after the postures as you would with a normal exercise routine. Emptying the bowels before starting is also recommended.

13. **If you have any pre-existing medical or health condition, please consult the contra-indications listed for each posture as well as discussing with a physician or qualified guide before undertaking the postures.**

14. **Stop practice if there is excessive pain in any area of the body. Please use common sense and sensitivity to your own body when performing the postures.**

15. Practice regularly. It is best to setup a routine, whether it is three times a week or everyday or during the weekends. A regular time is also beneficial as it trains the body and mind to expect and accept the routine -- cultivating a good habit.

# Healing Postures of the 18 Siddhas

Relaxation, Rejuvenation, and Connection with Immortal Guides of Humanity

# Tirumular (Sundarnath)

A very advanced yogi called Sundarnath came down from the Himalayas and was travelling through southern India when he came across some cows crying piteously in a meadow. Going closer to investigate, he saw a dead cow-herd lying by a tree. He tried to encourage the cows to leave and go back to their home but they were too attached to the dead man. Finally, in his compassion, Sundarnath used his yogic powers to enter the dead body so that the cowherd appeared to live again. After carefully hiding his real body, he prodded the cows away and they obediently began to go home. He followed them to the village where they came from. The villagers greeted him and he found out his name was Mular. When he came to his home, Mular's wife scolded him for being so late. As soon as he could, he slipped away and ran back to the grazing meadow but was surprised to find that his real body was not in the hiding place. He realized immediately that Lord Shiva, the Lord of all Yogis, had taken his body away and he had to stay in Mular's body to teach yoga to the people of Southern India.

He became known far and wide for his great yogic knowledge and authored the greatest yogic compendium in the Tamil language. Since he became known as Tirumular, his treatise is called Tirumandirum. After many years, he found his body and returned to the Himalayas.

According to Tirumular, *"Those who live in yoga and see the divine light and power through yoga are the siddhars or perfect humans."*

> *To them who speak of Hara's holy feet and weep*
> *To them who daily contemplate the Great One's might feet*
> *To them who, fixed in deep devotion, await to serve,*
> *To them the Eternal's all-filling Grace comes.*
>    *Sutra 40, Tirumandirum*

Posture 1

# Salutation to Divine

## Benefits:

Energetic: Stimulates and awakens the Crown Chakra at the top of the head

Mental / Spiritual: Promotes humility

Physical: rejuvenates the glandular system; improves low blood pressure

Therapeutic: for those suffering from lumbar lordosis

**Avoid this posture: those with prolapsed disc, commonly called a collapsed spinal disc or slipped disc**

**Affirmation used during holding phase: Om Kriya Babaji Nama Aum**

Sanskrit Name: Atma Namaskar

Siddha: Tirumular (Sundarnath)

The sacred salutation **Om Kriya Babaji Nama Aum** is used in this and the following posture to bow to the Divine within us, that is our True Self. *Om* is the source of all creation; *Kriya* is action with awareness; *Babaji* is the immortal Being from whom flows all evolutionary impulse and practice; *Nama* means salutation and *Aum* is the sound of the universe within.

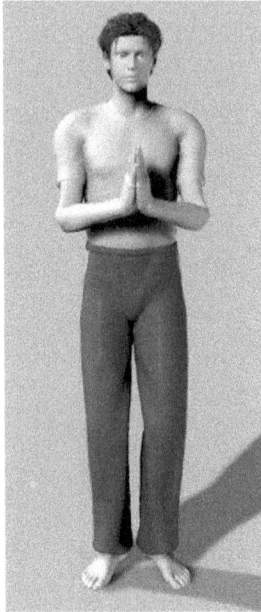

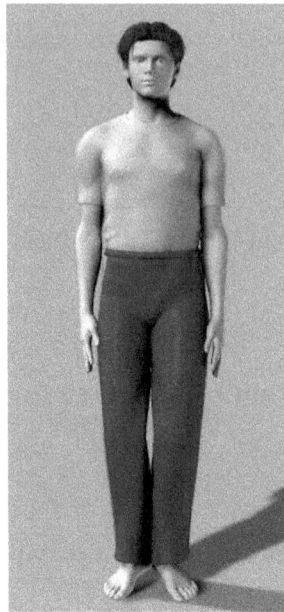

Stand erect with heels together and toes apart; the palms of the hands are placed together at the heart level - this position is called *namaskara* or *anjali mudra* - we bow to the Divine within us. lower the hands by the sides; shoulders and legs relaxed; eyes softly focused ahead. This is an open and receptive pose; all tension is released.

Kneel down with body still erect from head to knees; keep hands by the sides; knees and feet should be together.

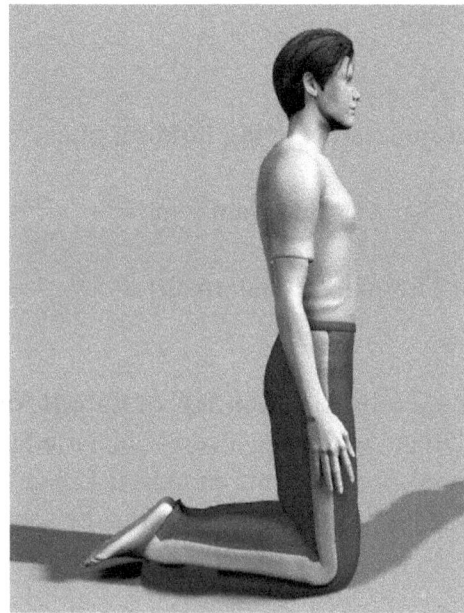

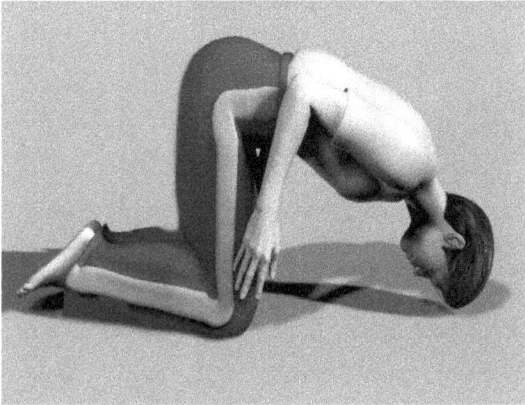

Move the head forward and place the crown of the head on the floor; hands still at the sides.

Move hands forward in front of the head and place the palms together.

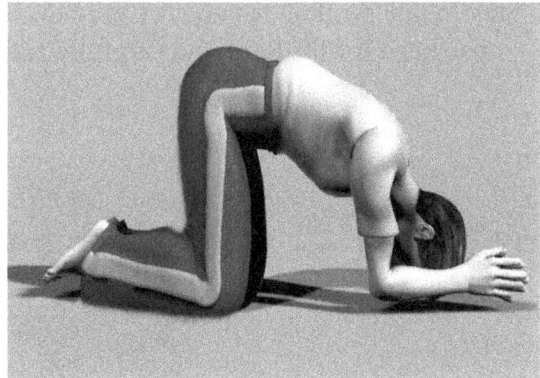

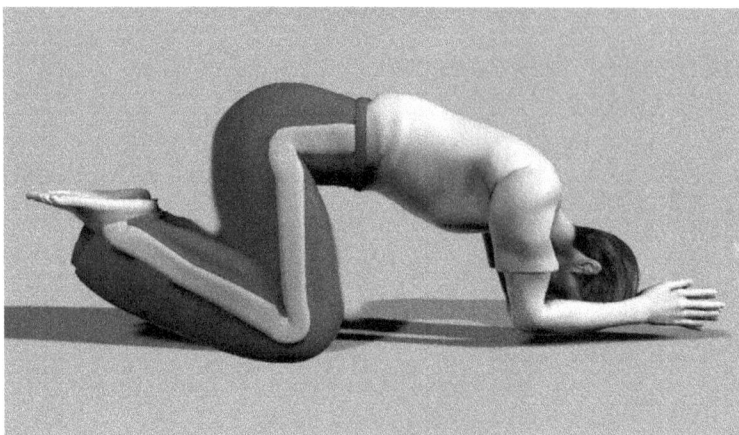

Raise the feet up off the floor; balancing on knees, forearms and head.

Keep breathing normally and chant aloud,"Om Kriya Babaji Nama Aum."

Stay in this position for about 1 minute.  Then lower the feet; move hands back to the sides; raise head off the floor and carefully stand up in the beginning pose with palms together.

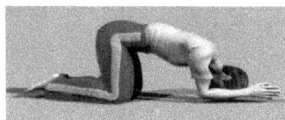

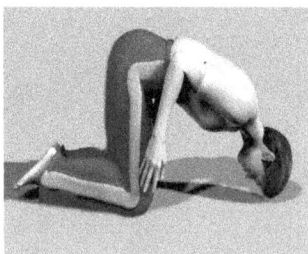

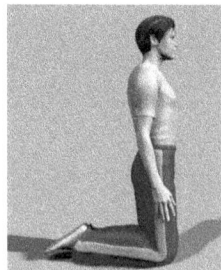

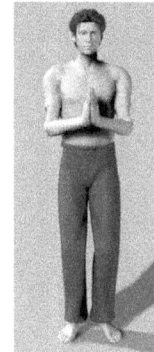

Relax and let go of all tensions in the body and mind.

# Valmiki

The Rishi Valmiki who authored the epic Ramayana started out as a robber who preyed upon travellers in the forest. He once tried to rob a great sage who instead robbed him of his negativity and he fell at the feet of the sage and asked for salvation. When the sage attempted to give him the mantra of Rama, Valmiki felt unworthy and so the sage told him to repeat, "ma-ra, ma-ra" which means "die,die." As Valmiki continuously repeated the sage's sacred words of holy vibration, it became "ra-ma, ra-ma," the name of the Lord incarnated on Earth.

For a very long time, Valmiki continued his meditation - so long that an anthill formed around him. In time, the sage came back and called him to appear and the transformed robber came out of the anthill (valmiki) and therefore he was given the name of Valmiki.

Once Valmiki came upon a hunter who had killed two birds in love-play. This is considered a heinous crime and Valmiki spontaneously sang out a curse in a new musical metre called Anushtubh. The divine sage musician Narada heard it and blessed Valmiki to compose the Ramayana in the new metre.

It is not clear whether the siddha Valmiki (also called Vanihar) is the same as the Rishi Valmiki, but tradition holds this to be the case.

According to the book "Valmiki Suthira Gyanam" authored by Siddhar Valmiki, "*By purifying the mind and attaining perfection one becomes a siddha (Tamil Chittan); He is indeed fit to be called Shiva.*"

# Salutation to the Sun

## Benefits:

Energetic: Stimulates all chakras and recharges with prana or life-force energy

Mental / Spiritual: Connects with the Divine within and without.

Physical: stretches and exercises the entire body

Therapeutic: for stiffness and lethargy

**Mantra used: Om Kriya Babaji Nama Aum**

Sanskrit Name: Surya Namaskar

Siddha: Valmiki

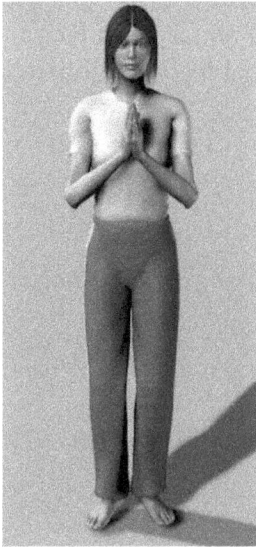

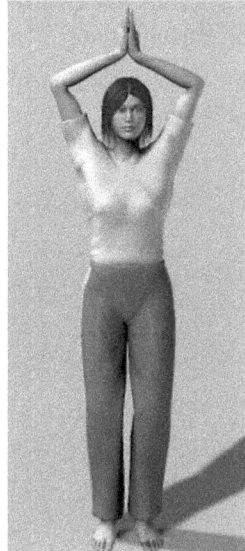

Stand with heels together and toes apart, palms joined together at the heart level. Slowly raise hands a few inches above the head keeping the palms together. Hold with normal breathing and repeat aloud, "Om Kriya Babaji Nama Aum." Feel the vibration of the sound at the top of the head.

Keeping the palms together, lower the hands to the level of the mid-brow. Repeat aloud,"Om Kriya Babaji Nama Aum," as you feel the vibration at the eyebrow center.

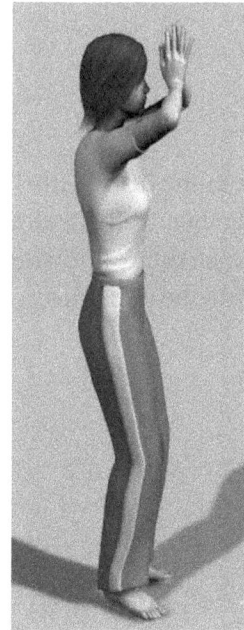

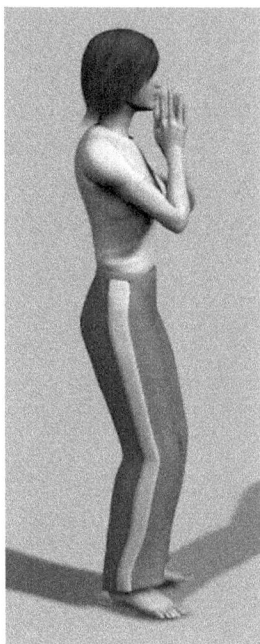

Still keeping the palms together, lower the hands to the throat center. Intone aloud, "Om Kriya Babaji Nama Aum," and feel the vibration at the throat.

Lower the hands to the heart center while keeping the palms together. Repeat aloud, "Om Kriya Babaji Nama Aum," allowing the vibration to permeate the heart center.

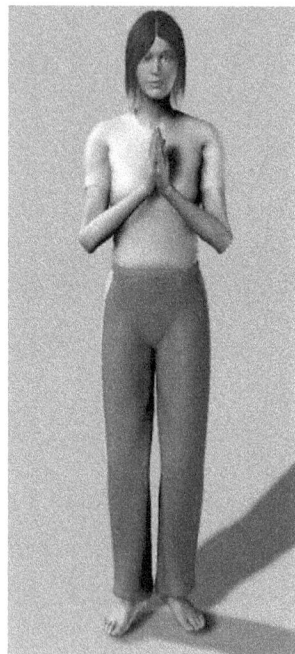

16

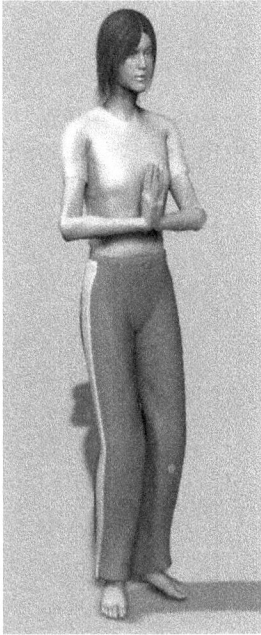

Keep the palms together as much as possible as you lower the hands to the level of the navel. Repeat, "Om Kriya Babaji Nama Aum." and feel the vibration at the navel center.

Move the left leg forward a few inches and lower the left knee to the floor as you lower the right knee close to the left. Raise the palms to the top of the head.

Repeat, " Om Kriya Babaji Nama Aum."

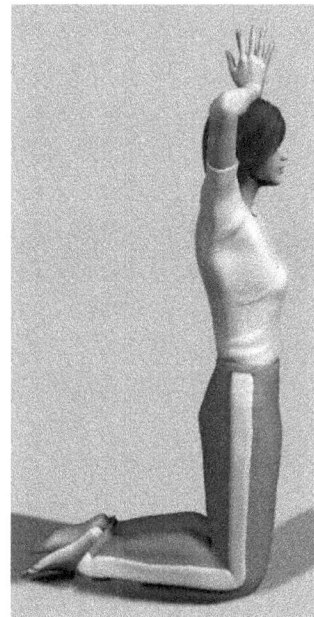

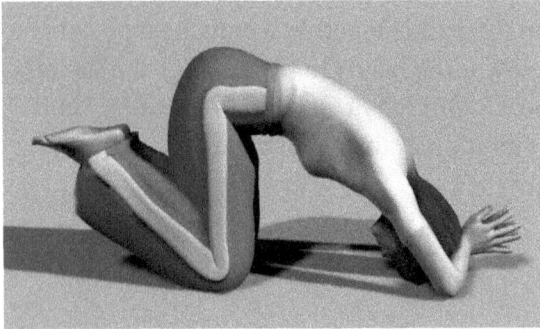

Lower head to the floor, keeping the palms together on top of the head. Raise feet of the floor -- salutation to the Divine.
Repeat, "Om Kriya Babaji Nama Aum."

Lower feet to floor. Place hands by the side of the knees and raise head off the floor. Move right knee forward between hands and stretch left leg backwards; the back is arched and the tops of the feet lie as flat as possible on the floor. Look upwards and repeat, "Om Kriya Babaji Nama Aum."

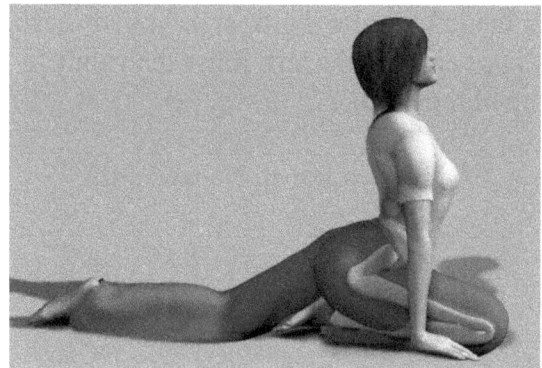

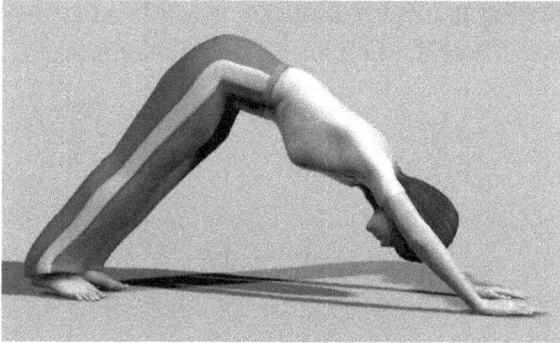

Move right leg back and keep both feet together. Slide palms forward. Arch hips up and lower head down. Repeat, "Om Kriya Babaji Nama Aum."

Lower hips to the floor, keeping the feet together. Arch back and look upwards. Repeat, "Om Kriya Babaji Nama Aum."

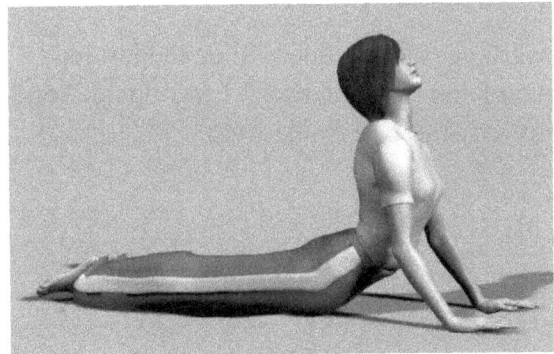

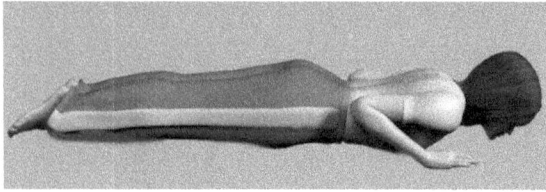

Keeping palms on the floor, lower head to the floor. Repeat, "Om Kriya Babaji Nama Aum."

Repeat movements from the previous postures in reverse order. Raise hips off the floor and look up. Repeat, "Om Kriya Babaji Nama Aum."

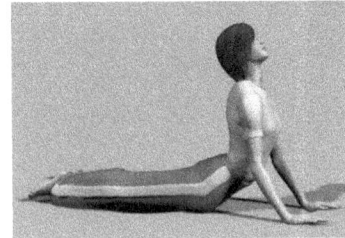

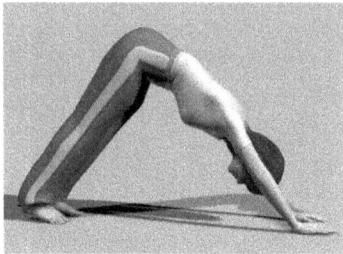

Keeping feet together, arch back and lower head towards floor. Repeat, "Om Kriya Babaji Nama Aum."

Lower knees to the floor. Slide the left leg forward and right leg back. Look up and repeat, "Om Kriya Babaji Nama Aum."

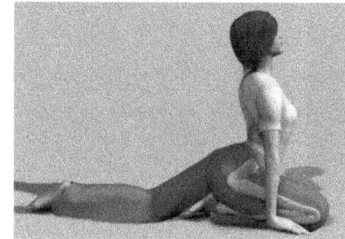

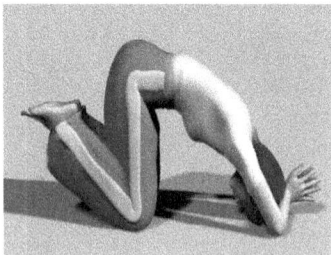

Move right leg forward, keeping both feet together. Raise palms together over head and lowever head to the floor. Raise feet off floor. Repeat, "Om Kriya Babaji Nama Aum."

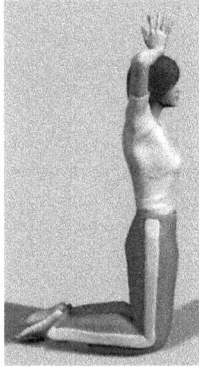

Lower feet to the floor and raise head from the floor. Repeat, "Om Kriya Babaji Nama Aum."

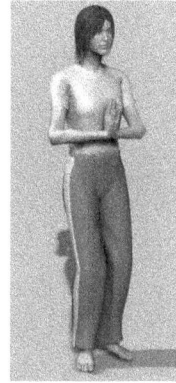

Lower palms to the navel and feet the vibration as you repeat, "Om Kriya Babaji Nama Aum."

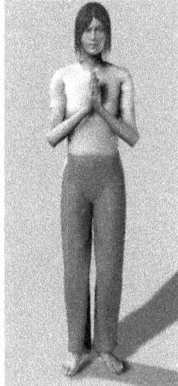

Raise palms to the heart level and feel vibration there as you repeat, "Om Kriya Babaji Nama Aum."

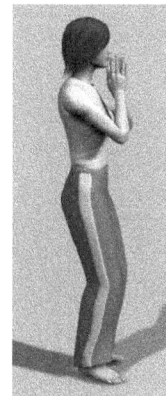

Raise palms to the throat level and feel the vibration as you repeat, "Om Kriya Babaji Nama Aum."

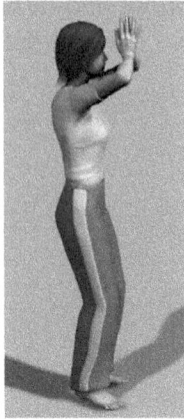

Raise palms to the mid-eyebrow level and feel the vibration there as you repeat, "Om Kriya Babaji Nama Aum."

Raise the palms up above the head and feel the vibration as you intone, "Om Kriya Babaji Nama Aum."

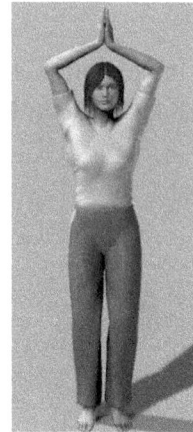

Turn clockwise and chant to the Divine Light, exposing yourself to the sunlight if possible. The physical and sublte bodies are magnetized and cleansed by this invocation, while the aura is strengthened.

## Chant to the Divine Light

| | |
|---|---|
| Deepam Jyoti Parabrahman | I bow to the Light of Supreme |
| Deepam Sarvam Tamobagam | I take refuge in Divine Grace |
| Deepanay Sathyathey Sarvam | All is done by that Truth |
| | |
| Nyarua Deepam Namosthuthey | Salutations to the Sun |
| Kaalai Deepam Namosthuthey | Salutations to the Light of the morning |
| Ucchi Deepam Namosthuthey | Salutations to the Light of Midday |
| Santhyaa Deepam Namosthuthey | Salutations to the Light of Evening |
| Nisi Deepam Namosthuthey | Salutations to the Light of Night |
| | |
| Anbu Deepam Nomosthuthey | Salutations to Divine Love |
| Ahimsa Deepam Nomosthuthey | Salutations to Non-violence |
| Asana Deepam Nomosthuthey | Salutations to rejuvenating postures |
| Prana Deepam Nomosthuthey | Salutations to mastery of Breath |
| Dhyana Deepam Namosthuthey | Salutations to mastery of Mind |
| Jnana Deepam Namosthuthey | Salutations to Wisdom |
| Mantra Deepam Namosthuthey | Salutations to Sacred Sound |
| Bhakti Deepam Namosthuthey | Salutations to Devotion to the Divine |
| | |
| Babaji Deepam Namosthuthey | Salutations to Immortal Babaji |
| Annai Deepam Namosthuthey | Salutations to Mataji |
| Amman Deepam Namosthuthey | Salutations to Discipleship |
| Yoga Deepam Namosthuthey | Salutations to Yoga |

# Kudambai

Once there was a woman who had a great desire for a daughter but instead was blessed with a baby boy. She nonetheless treated her son as a baby girl, dressing him in girl's clothing and putting earings on his ears. Other people also started seeing him as a girl and calling him kudambai which means ear-rings. The boy was born with great wisdom and even after achieving the divine state of a siddha, he was known as Kudambai Siddha.

There is also a correlation between ear-rings and the coiled potential energy called Kundalini, as many siddhas pierce the cartilage of their ears and wore ear-rings to facilitate the flow and control the "serpent power."

In his poems, the Siddha says:

*Will the amassed wealth go with you,*
        *at the time of death, kudambay?*
        *Will they go with you.*

*Even if you can grasp the entire world,*
        *not an atom of dust can follow you, kudambay*
        *not an atom of dust can follow you.*

*Relatives, near and dear ones, siblings,*
        *parents and children - will they remain your companions, kudambay?*
        *Will they stay your companions?*

*Only deeds, both good and bad, even discreetly done*
        *definitely will go with the doer, kudambay!*
        *definitley will go with the doer.*

Posture 3

# Shoulder Stand

## Benefits:

Energetic: throat chakra or fifth energy center

Mental / Spiritual: promotes intuition

Physical: stimulate the thryroid gland and improve eye-sight

Therapeutic: improved circulation; headache, chest colds

**Avoid this posture: those with high-blood pressure; slipped cervical vertebrae**

**Affirmation used during holding phase: Divine Peace floods my body, mind and soul**

Sanskrit Name: Sarvangasana

Siddha: Kudumbai

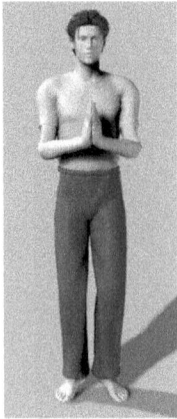

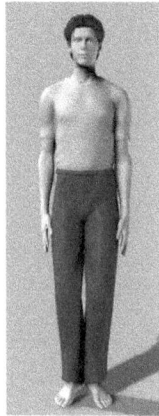

Stand erect with heels together and toes apart; the palms of the hands are placed together at the heart level. Lower the hands by the sides; shoulders and legs relaxed; eyes softly focused ahead.

Lie down on the back.

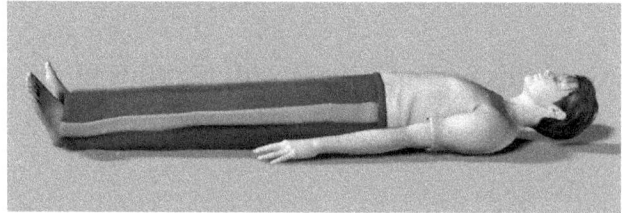

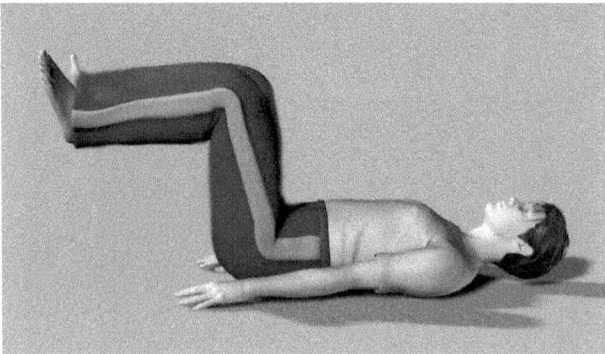

Raise the feet off the floor while keeping the knees bent. Flex the toes and circle the feet.

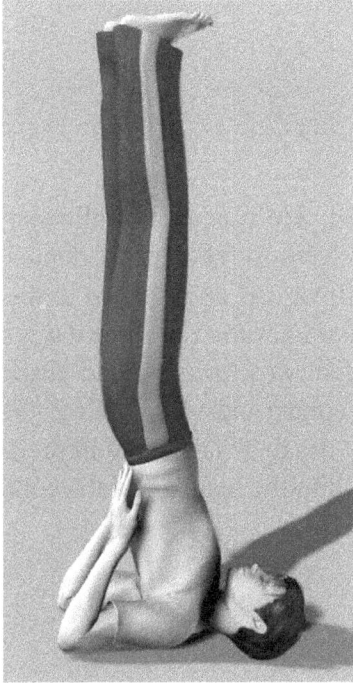

Press down with your palms on the floor; hold the abdominal muscules. Straighten the spine; raising the legs vertical so that the pelvis is directly above the shoulders. Place the hands at the lower back for support. Press the sternum against the chin to create chin lock with the chin touching the hollow of the throat. Bring the elbows together to form a triangle and protect the head and shoulders. Hold this posture focusing on the throat for a miniumum of 1 minute and upto 3 minutes. **Repeat the affirmation mentally, "Divine Peace floods my body, mind and soul."**

Bend and lower the knees towards the head. Place palms on floor. Lower legs to the floor and relax for about 1 minute. Raise hands over head, stretch and sit up. Lower hands to touch toes; stand up with palms together.

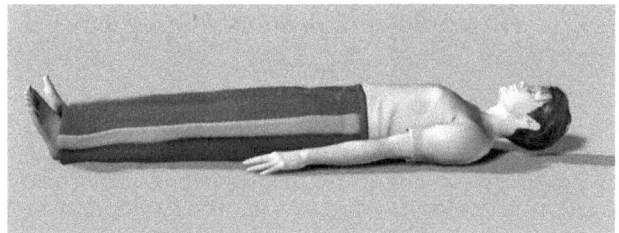

# Matsyendranath

A yogi was meditating on a boat and in a storm, fell into the sea. He was then swallowed by a great fish, but he stayed in his meditative state throughout. The fish went to the deepest depths of the sea attracted by the still state there. It so happened that the Lord Shiva had come down to the bottommost part to reveal the highest secrets of yoga to his Shakti, the Goddess Parvati. For three days, Lord Shiva gave instructions, Unbeknownest to Him, the yogi inside the fish was listening and absorbing these greatest of teachings. After three days, Lord Shiva finishes his discourse and asked Lady Parvati whether She had understood everything. Both the Lady and the "yogi in the fish" answered in the affirmative. Lord Shiva smiled and liberated the yogi from the fish and gave him the name of Matsyendranath - the Lord of Fish.

In the Karana Jnanam, the Mahasiddha says:

*Discarding the ego-desire*
      *absorbing the sacred scriptures*
*Mind-restrained and wholly united with wisdom*
      *conjoining with the attributeless One*
*Perceiving the secret source of motion in space*
      *lost in union with "that"*
*Detached from duality*
      *He is said to be achored in wisdom.*
             *verse 10*

# Fish Pose

## Benefits:

Energetic: activating the pituitary and pineal glands

Mental / Spiritual: stimulates the third eye

Physical: removes lethargy; improved spinal vertebrae

Therapeutic: kyphosis (hunchback)

**Avoid this posture: pregnancy; spinal bifida; heart disease**

**Affirmation used during holding phase: Divine Light fills my body, mind and soul**

Sanskrit Name: Matsyasana

Siddha: Matsyendranath

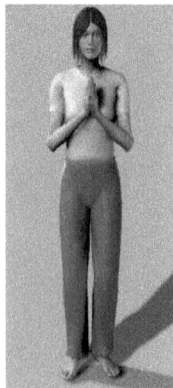

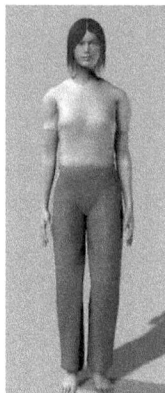

Stand erect with heels together and toes apart; the palms of the hands are placed together at the heart level. Lower the hands by the sides; shoulders and legs relaxed; eyes softly focused ahead.

Sit down crossing the right leg in front. Place the right foot on the left thigh. Push the right knee up and down to loosen the knee.

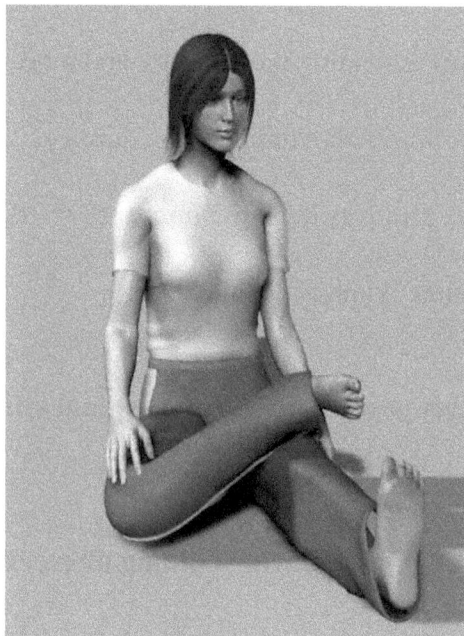

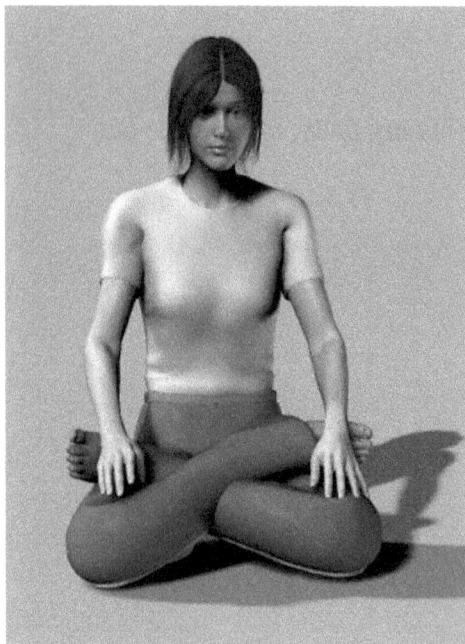

Place the left foot on the right thigh; push left knee up and down. Keep feet crossed in the lotus position.

If the knees are too stiff for the lotus, keep the legs crossed in a simple postures.

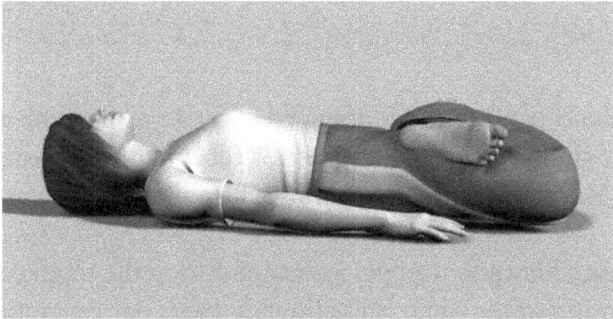

Bend forwards, holding onto the knees. Roll onto back; lower hands and knees to floor.

Us the elbows to support yourself. Raise the head and shoulders off the floor. Lower the head to the floor, arching the back. Place the hands on the thighs so that the top of the head is on the floor. Hold for about a minute, breathing normally. **Repeat the affirmation, "Divine Light fills my body, mind and soul."**

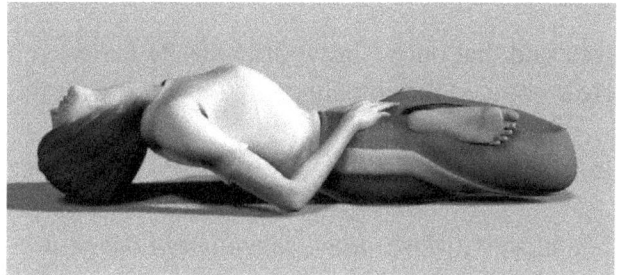

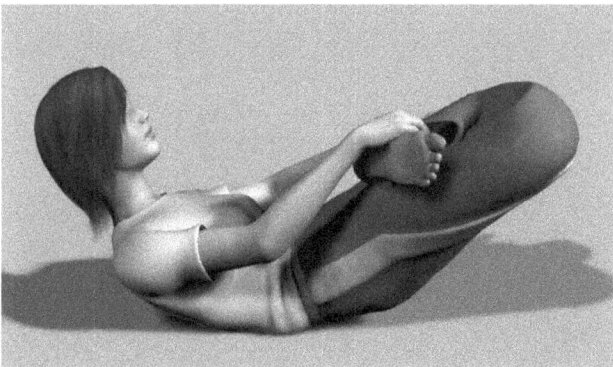

Lower elbows to the floor and raise the head off the floor. Lower back to the floor. Raise the knees off the floor and hold the feet with the hands. Rock forwards and roll backwards on the back at least seven times with tightened abdominal muscles and chin tucked in. Sit up and straighten the legs, flex them and relax.

# Karuvoorar

A brahmin by birth, he become a disciple of the Siddha Boganath and renounced his caste to become a siddha.  This is because a distinctive feature of the siddhas is that they do not recognize the caste system and came from all walks of life. He was called Karuvoorar after the name of his village, Karuvur.

He achieved great fame during the construction of Brahadiswarar Temple in Tanjur during the reign of Rajaraja Chola. There was difficulty with the installation of the giant Shivalinga in the inner sanctum and the King was advised by the astral form of Boganath to secure the help of Karuvoorar.
The siddha successfully installed the giant linga as well as raising and affixing the eighty-ton capstone to the top of the 225 foot high gate-tower (gopuram) - mighty engineering feats.

It is said that once Karuvoorar was be harassed by the brahmins and took refuge in the Shiva temple. He embraced the shivalinga and merged with the Divine.

In his poems, Karuvoorar emphasizes experience over mere learning of scriptures:

*The memory of one life is forgotten in the next*
*        Consequently, one does not realize the truth.*
*If one relies on the written words of scriptures, will the thirst for reality be satisfied?*
*        Is hunger appeased by looking at the cooking vessels?*

Posture 5

# Standing Crane

## Benefits:

Energetic: stimulates base and third-eye energy centers

Mental / Spiritual: flexiibility and tolerance

Physical: improves digestion

Therapeutic: diabetes; osteoporosis; vertebral osteoarthritis

**Avoid this posture: heart disease; sciatica; high blood pressure; abdominal hernia**

**Affirmation used during holding phase: My Being expands into infinite space**

Sanskrit Name: Nindra Kokkuasana

Siddha: Karuvoorar

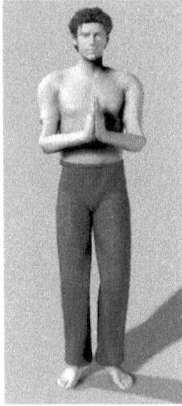

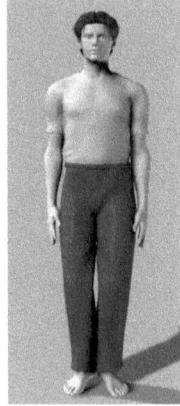

Stand erect with heels together and toes apart; the palms of the hands are placed together at the heart level. Lower the hands by the sides; shoulders and legs relaxed; eyes softly focused ahead.

Stretch hands above head.

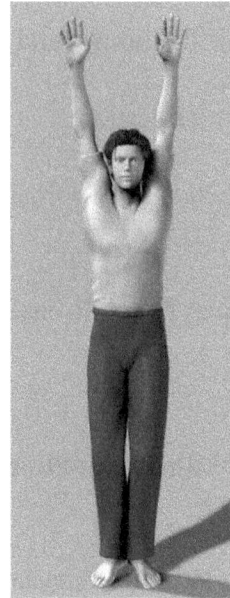

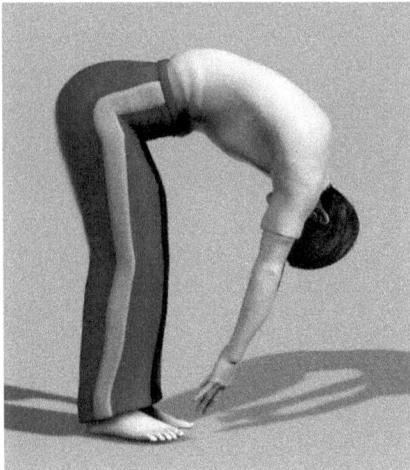

Bend forwards at the hips, pausing halfway with hands parallel to the floor. Stretch arms forward to flatten the back. Let the head and hands drop gently, lowering the fingertips as near to the floor as possible.

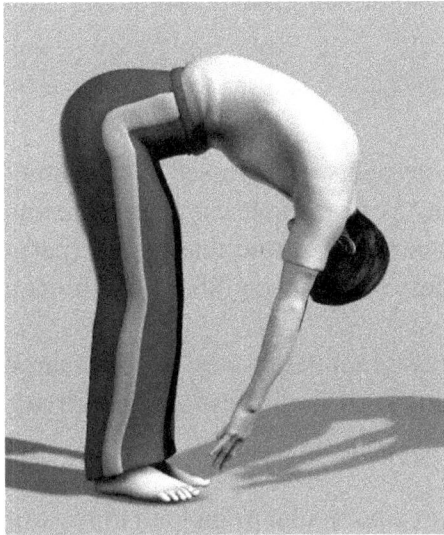

With micro-movements, gently move up and down focusing on the abdomen.

Stop the movement and bend the knees deeply. Bring your chest against the thighs. Hold the ankles or back of legs. Breathe into the stretch. Press into heels and lift the hips while slowly straighten the legs as far as comfortable. Keep the chest against the thighs.

**Hold position for a minute and repeat the affirmation, "My Being expands into infinite space."**

Let go of the ankles. Slowly roll upright, one vertebrae at a time, bringing the arms up and reaching them up above the head. Release hands back down to the sides. Relax for a minute and then place palms together at the heart level.

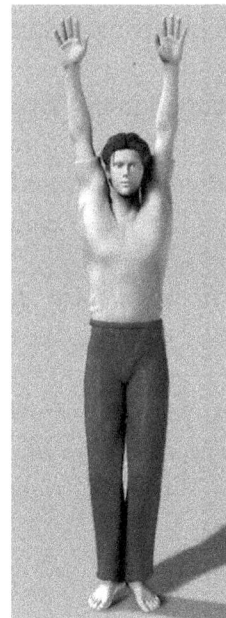

# Patanjali

Once upon a time, Ananta the thousand headed king of the serpents was blessed by a vision of Lord Shiva. He immediately acquired a great aspiration to become a yogi and to teach Yoga to humanity. He asked Lord Vishnu and was granted a boon to incarnate on earth. It is said that he fell (pat) into the palms (anjali) of a virtuous woman called Gonika and manifested as her son. She called him Patanjali.

According to Indian Tradition, the sage Patanjali was a famous grammarian who wrote a learned commentary on Panini's tome of Sanskrit Grammar ( Ashta-Adhyayi or Eight Lessons), and lived around 2nd Century BC.

Patanjali is more remembered and revered for his summary of a particular Yoga Path in his work Yoga Darshana which is popularly called the Yoga Sutras. This is a compilation and systemization of a philosophy of Yoga which was heretofore kept hidden. From this work onwards, Yoga was seen to have a solid philosophical base and competed with other schools of philosophy. In this respect, a word of caution is in order — philosophy in the Indian context always denoted a course of action and a way of life, rather than a purely academic pursuit as it has become in the West.

According to Patanjali in his Yoga Sutras:

*When the fluctuations in the mind-stuff are completely restricted, then the state of Yoga is attained.*
          *Pada 1, sutra 2*

*Posture is that which is steady, stable and firm as well as easy and pleasant.*
          *Pada 2, sutra 46*

*Postures are important for releasing tension, producing relaxation and a favorable physical environment for mind to identify with the Universal Consciousness.*
          *Pada 2, sutra 47*

# Bow Pose

## Benefits:

Energetic: stimulates navel center

Mental / Spiritual: self-control

Physical: strengthening of digestive system

Therapeutic: diabetes; gastrointestinal disorders; menstrual disorders; obesity

**Avoid this posture: high blood pressure; heart disease; colitis; peptic or duodenal ulcers**

**Affirmation used during holding phase: My energies and emotions are completely under control**

Sanskrit Name: Dhanurasana

Siddha: Patanjali

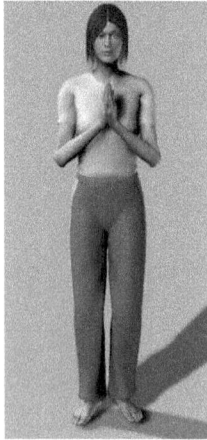

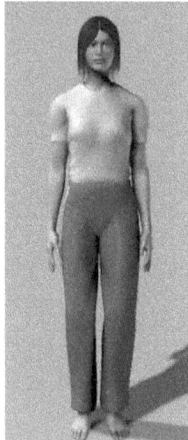

Stand erect with heels together and toes apart; the palms of the hands are placed together at the heart level. Lower the hands by the sides; shoulders and legs relaxed; eyes softly focused ahead.

Lie down on your front with hands by the side. Keep the legs together.

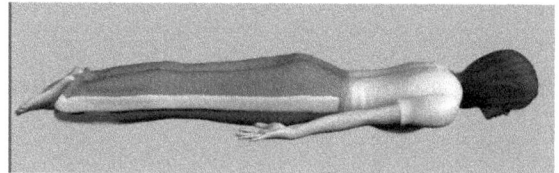

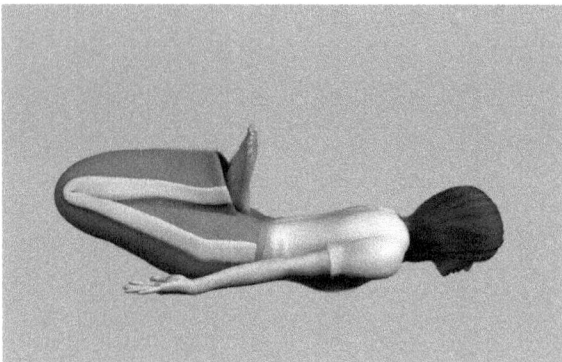

Fold your knees and bring the feet to the buttocks, in effect kicking the buttocks if possible. Do this motion for about a dozen times.

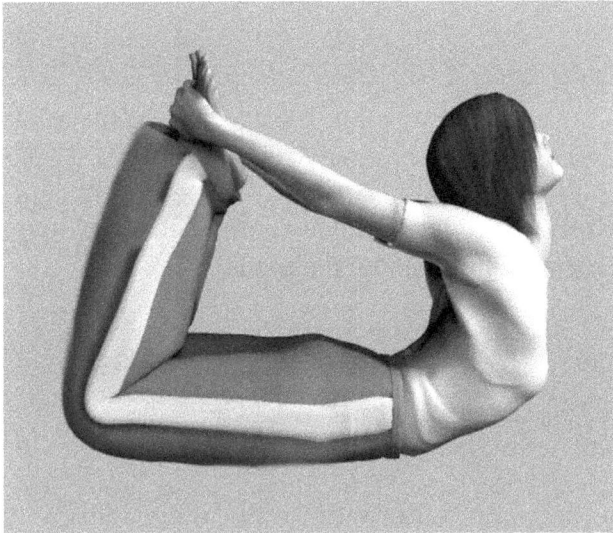

Stop the motion and grab your feet with your hands. Press feet backward, lifting the head and shoulders upward and then lift up the thighs, arching backwards. Hold this position for about 30 seconds, while repeating **the affirmation, "My energies and emotions are completely under control."**

Then begin rocking motion forwards and backwards. Do this rocking for about dozen times. Stop motion, lower back, keeping hands on feet.

Once again, pull up with arched back. Roll to left side.

*If this is difficult, you may wish to cross your arms on the back when your roll to the side.*

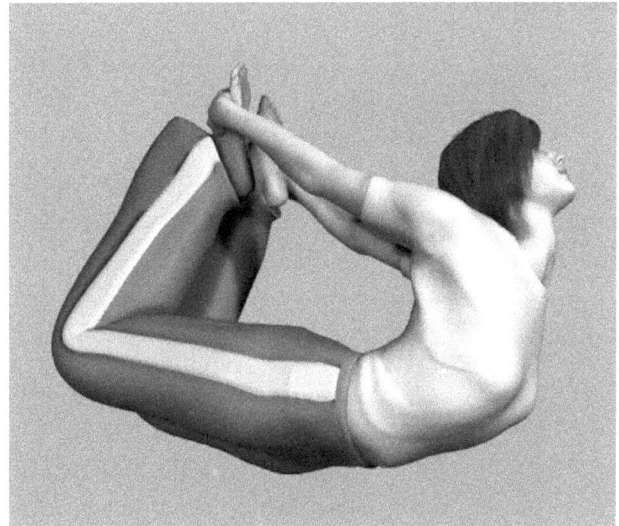

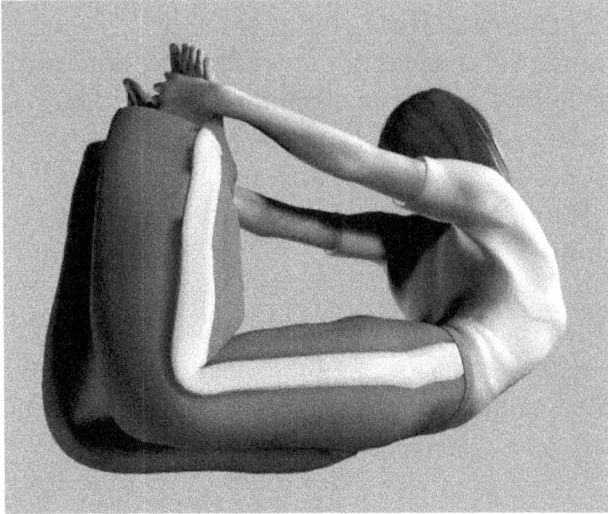

Roll to the other side and continue this side to side motion for about ten times.

Stop motion and return to the center. Relax in this position.

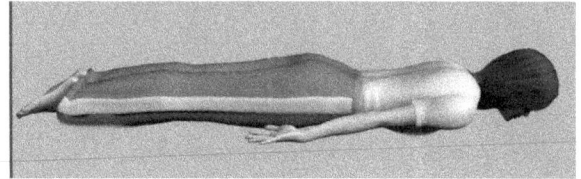

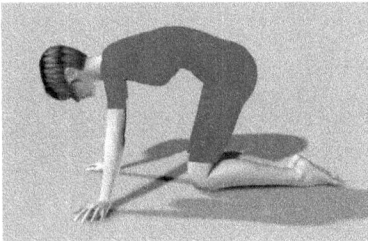

When ready to get up, sit up on hands and knees and perform a few cat stretches. Then sit on your heels stretching the hands in front in a dog stretch and finally rising into the downward dog. Walk towards the hands and stand up with palms together.

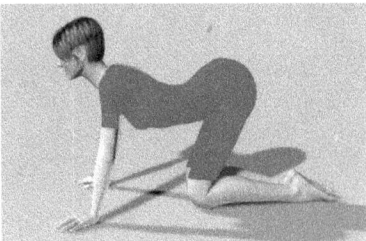

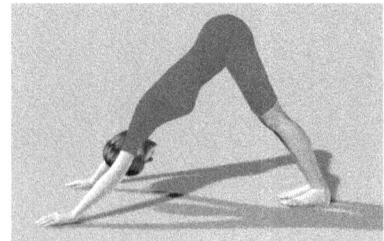

# Bhoganath

There are many legends about Bogar. One connects him with Kashi or Banares in Northern India.He demonstrated miraculous powers as well as Divine knowledge of Siddha Sciences. In South India, it is said that Bhogar belonged to the caste of goldsmiths, and became a Siddha under the guidance of Kalanginath from the Nath Tradition. In Bogar's Saptakanda he reveals details of various medicinal preparations to his disciple Pullippani (so named as he is believed to have wandered in the forests atop a puli or tiger) and at every stage he quotes his guru as the authority.

Bhogar was a great devotee of Muruga, a son of Lord Shiva. He spent many years in Palani, a great shrine to Lord Muruga. There is a temple dedicated to Boganath in Palani. In it is a figure made by him and enhanced by a mixture of nine poisonous herbs and minerals which when combined gave rise to healing properties.

Under the direction of his Guru, Bhogar proceeded to China to spread the knowledge of siddha sciences and he may have some relationship with Boyang or even Laotse, the author of the Tao Teh King, a taoist classic. Just as with Sundarnath, it is possible that Bhoganath may have taken on a new body - a Chinese body. He evidently brought the science of immortality to China.

Even to this day, Bhoganath is still said to inspire and help those devoted to innovation and the sciences. He has promised that the practice of Siddha Yoga can bestow immortality:

> *For liberation from rebirth, direct the life-force to the energy centers*
> *There Kundalini is the Guru, Whose wisdom will remove suffering*
> *Whose Divine Nectar trickling down will give peace of mind.*
> *Verse 3, Samadhi Diksai-10*

Posture 7

# Topsy Turvy Pose

## Benefits:

Energetic: stimulates the heart center

Mental / Spiritual: equilibrium - centering

Physical: strengthens the heart; removes toxins

Therapeutic: hypertension; emphysema; bronchitis


**Avoid this posture: high blood pressure; enlarged thyroid; prolapsed disc**


**Affirmation used: My body is filled with the Divine nectar of rejuvenation**


Sanskrit Name: Vibareetha Karani asana

Siddha: Bhoganath

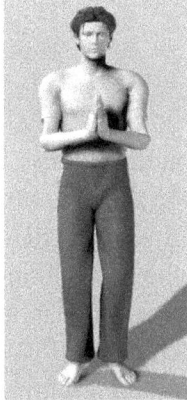

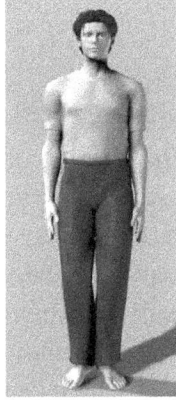

Stand erect with heels together and toes apart; the palms of the hands are placed together at the heart level. Lower the hands by the sides; shoulders and legs relaxed; eyes softly focused ahead.

Lie down on your back with hands by the side.

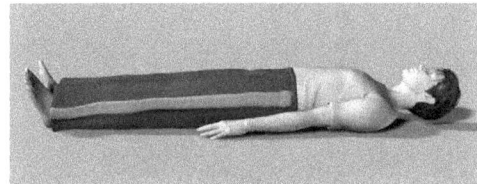

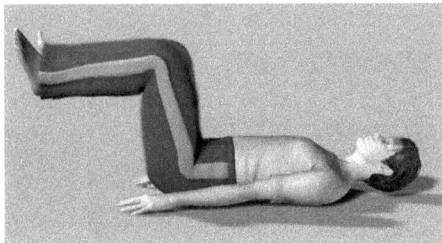

Raise knees off the floor, keeping the feet on the floor. Then raise the feet off the floor keeping the lower leg parallel to the floor. Wriggle the toes and rotate the feet.

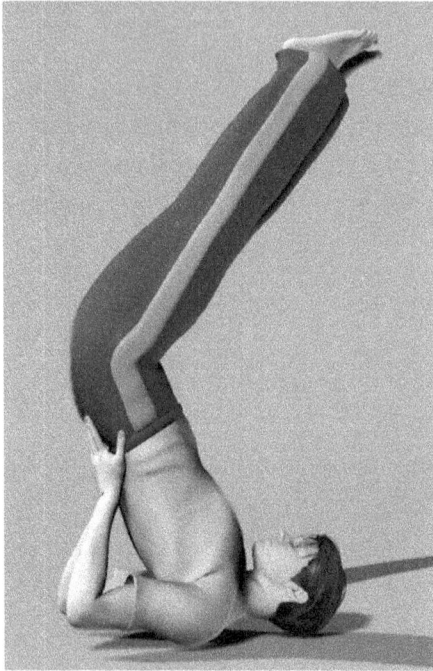

Press down with your hands on the floor to lift the legs up. Bring your hands to the hips to support the legs, keeping the elbows on the floor close together. The weight of the body should rest evenly between the elbows and the shoulders. The chin should not touch the hollow of the neck . The legs should be tilted slightly over the head. Hold this position for about 1 minute and even 3 minutes. **Repeat the affirmation, "My body is filled with the Divine nectar of rejuvenation."**

*You can also do this next to the wall and rest the feet against the wall to hold for longer periods of time.*

Lower the knees closer to the head and then place the hands on the floor.  Lower the body in stages and relax.

Then raise your hands over your head; stretch. Sit up and touch your hands to your legs. Stand up with palms together at the heart level.

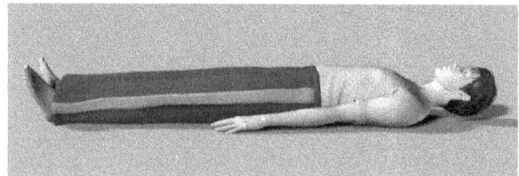

# Kamalamuni

This Siddha is very mysterious and is little of known of his life. A few hints are given by Bhoganath in his writings. Kamalamuni is said to have achieved Self-Realization in Madurai and live in a cave on Mt. Kailash, the abode of Lord Shiva. He initiated Bhoga into some higher spiritual practices and so would be considered to be at the level of Bhoga's Guru, Kalanginath (or Kalagninath).

From Janana Chaitanyam-18:

> *Achieve Self-Realization through moon-kundalini*
> *Experience the sun-kundalini, experience the fire-kundalini*
> *The joining of devotion with life-force will produce perfection*
> *When glow appears in the throat center. and the tinkling sound is heard,*
> *then liberation is near.*
> *Concentrate on inspiration of life-force and perceive the world*
> *to seek the True Master.*

The Siddhas usually gave their teachings in their own technical language which needs to be learned and interpreted to glean their profound knowledge. The uninitiated will have great difficulty in penetrating their secrets.

# Half Fish Pose

## Benefits:

Energetic: stimulates the sacral center; for insomnia

Mental / Spiritual: positivity

Physical: removes lethargy; improved spinal vertebrae

Therapeutic:corrects kyphosis (hunchback); relieves sciatica strain

**Avoid this posture: none**

**Affirmation used during holding phase: Awaken me to thy Divine Light**

Sanskrit Name: Ardha Matsyasana

Siddha: Kamalamuni

*This is a substitute for those who cannot do the Fish Pose (posture #4).*

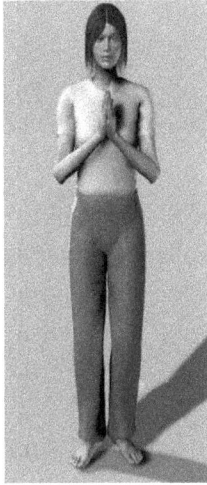

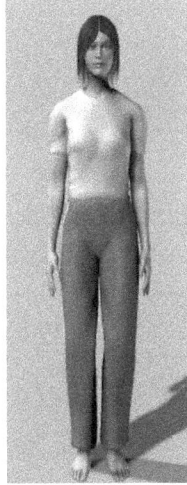

Stand erect with heels together and toes apart; the palms of the hands are placed together at the heart level. Lower the hands by the sides; shoulders and legs relaxed; eyes softly focused ahead.

Lie down on your back with arms by the side.

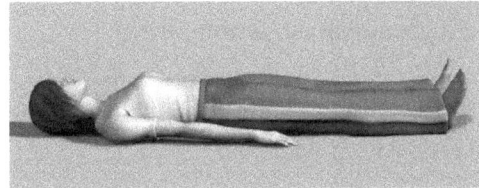

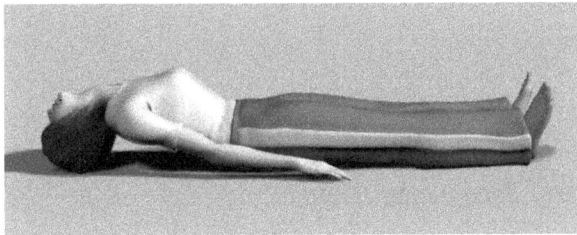

Press onto the forearms and using the elbows, lift the heart, arching the back, raise the head. Lower the head to the floor with the top of the head on the floor. Place the arms on the legs and open the feet, keeping the heels together. Stay in this position for about 1 minute with normal breathing. **Repeat the affirmation, "Awaken me to thy Divine Light."**

Relax by releasing the arms to the floor and using the elbows to support yourself. Lower the back to the floor and relax for a minute or so. Then raise your hands over your head; stretch. Sit up and touch your hands to your legs. Stand up with palms together at the heart level.

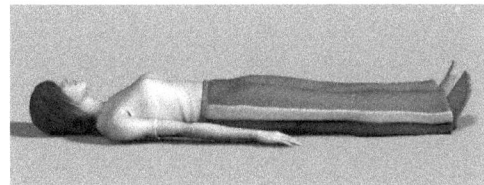

# Ramadeva

He was born Siddha who became a disciple of the sage Pulastya and devotee of Shiva-Shakti. In one of his works, he says, "*I achieved the supreme absorptive state of samadhi by the grace of the Guru and worship of Shiva-Shakti. When I was roaming all the eight directions, I realized the Divine Sound aspect of creation. She endowed me with everlasting Wisdom so that I regained my own essential nature.*"

Once while absorbed in samadhi in a coastal town of Tamil Nadu, he became aware of some Arab merchants and instantaneously reached Arabia. He took on Arab custom and was called Jacob and became a great teacher among them.

He wrote on many esoteric subjects, especially well-known is his work on Bija-mantras or sacred sounds.

> *My friend, don't get frustrated in the worship,*
> *Obtain the five aspects emanating from the Absolute;*
> *Without becoming, by grace, be!*
> *Evolve into the base, the crest and center, in the six centers;*
> *Disentangling oneself from ignorance,*
> *One should chant the emerging three letters of AUM.*
> *Even if the body expires, it will not die.*
> *The circle in the square and the central angel will become the triangle.*
>     *Verse 2 Pujavidhi-10*

# Plough Pose

## Benefits:

Energetic: stimulates the throat/neck chakra or energy center; control of sexual energy

Mental / Spiritual: discrimination

Physical: improve digestion, elimination and reproduction

Therapeutic: scoliosis (deviation of the vertebral column to one side)

**Avoid this posture: high blood pressure; hernia; slipped discs; sciatica; weakness of the cervical vertebrae**

**Affirmation used during the holding phase: New Life Awakens - Consciousness Expands**

Sanskrit Name: Halasana

Siddha: Ramadeva

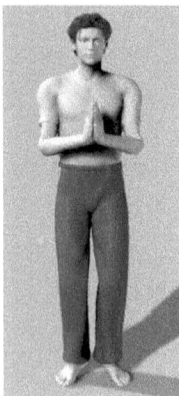

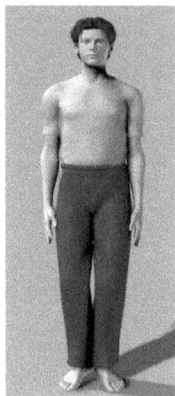

Stand erect with heels together and toes apart; the palms of the hands are placed together at the heart level. Lower the hands by the sides; shoulders and legs relaxed; eyes softly focused ahead.

Lie down on your back with hands by the side.

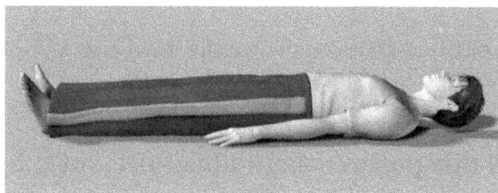

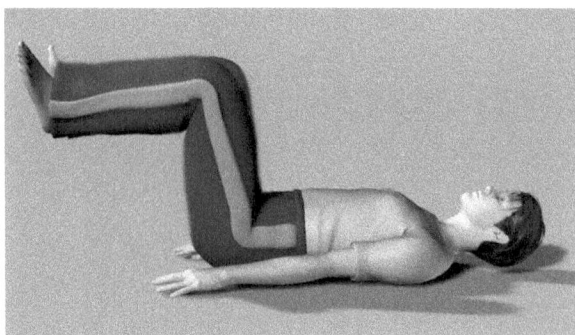

Raise legs up, keeping the seat on the floor. Press down with the hands and raise the legs straight up as in Shoulderstand (posture #2). To protect the neck, form a triangle between the head and shoulders by clasping the hands together and pulling the fists to the floor.

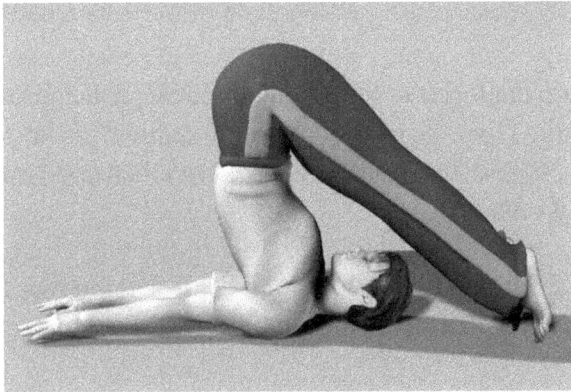

Slowly stretch the feet over the head as far as comfortable; keep the back straight; bring toes onto the floor. Rock the shoulders back and forth avoiding strain to the neck. Hold this for one or two minutes.

**Repeat the affirmation, "New Life Awakens - Consciousness Expands."**

Slowly lower knees to head. Unlock the hands and place them on the back to support yourself as you lower the legs slowly to the floor . Lie down relaxed for a minute or so.

Then raise your hands over your head; stretch. Sit up and touch your hands to your legs. Stand up with palms together at the heart level.

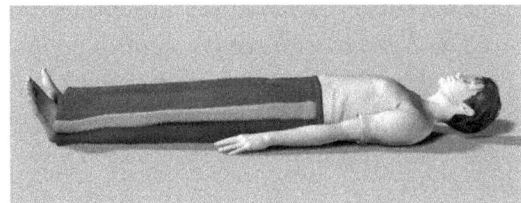

# Pambatti

He was a snake charmer by profession and once went into the forest to look for a mythical snake he had had heard about - it carried a priceless ruby in it's head. There he met Sattamuni, another of the 18 Siddhas who asked him what he was doing. When he explained, the Siddha laughed, and then cried out, "you keep that snake inside and you are searching for it outside?"

Sattamuni went on to explain, "There is a snake inside the body of all humans and it is known as kundalini. One who can control this snake is the true snake charmer. This snake carries a gem on its head - the gem called immortality."

Pambatti asked for initiation so that he could charm the snake within.

> *The everlasting bliss is ours.*
> *It is eternal and called liberation;*
> *Even while working, think of the Feet of the Primordial,*
> *And repeatedly sing and dance, Oh! Snake!*
> > *Verse 2*

> *Like oil is inseparable from the sesame,*
> *The Lord is with souls; meditate consciously*
> *On His Feet; and let your sincere devotion grow.*
> *And you, snake, dance with tranquility and humility.*
> > *Verse 4*

> *All the worldy riches like land, houses and others,*
> *Will they help you when the God of Death comes?*
> *What use are they when the body dies?*
> *Meditate on the feet of the Dancing God and dance, Oh! Snake!*
> > *Verse 40*

# Cobra Pose

## Benefits:

Energetic: stimulates the base chakra and third-eye center; connecting upper and lower energies

Mental / Spiritual: Determination

Physical: strengthens the reproductive system; removes toxins; opens and expands chest

Therapeutic: Thyroid disfunction

**Avoid this posture: pregnancy; chronic back pain; spinal bifida**

**Affirmation used during holding phase: I rise determinedly to overcome all obstacles**

Sanskrit Name: Bhujangasana

Siddha: Pambatti

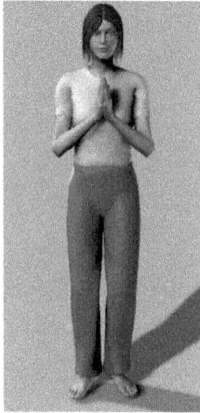

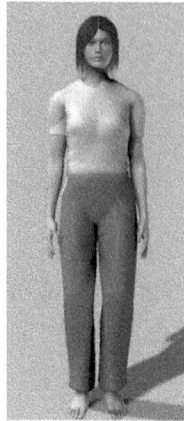

Stand erect with heels together and toes apart; the palms of the hands are placed together at the heart level. Lower the hands by the sides; shoulders and legs relaxed; eyes softly focused ahead.

Lie face down on the floor with hands by the side.

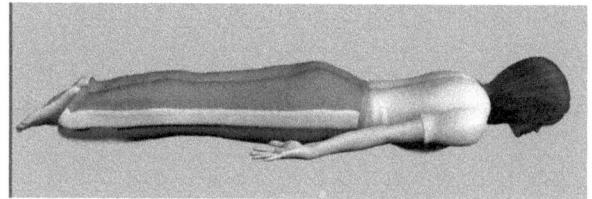

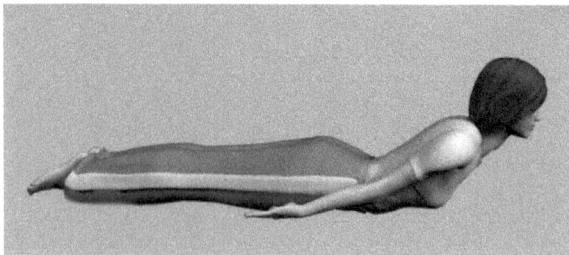

First variation: lift head, shoulders and torso, keeping hops on the floor. Repeat seven times.

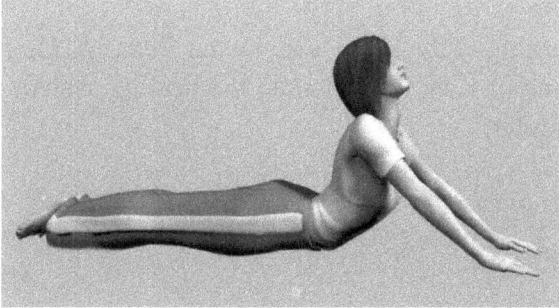

Second Variation: Place palms on the floor by the shoulders; slowly raise and arch the back, peeling yourself off the floor. Look up, keeping the hips on the floor. Lower shoulders and elbows by the chest. Hold for one minute, breathing normally. **Repeat the affirmation, "I rise determinedly to overcome all obstacles."**

Third variation: lower back and head. Stretch hands out in front of the head with palms together.; think of surrendering all mental disturbances. Arch back, raise head, stretch arms to side and sweep back, clapping hands together. Repeat seven times. Relax with hands stretched forward.

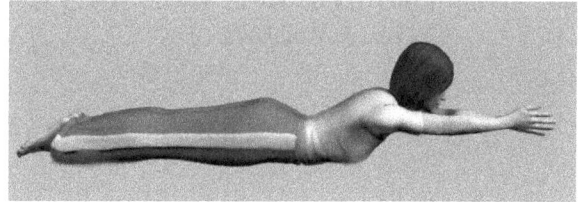

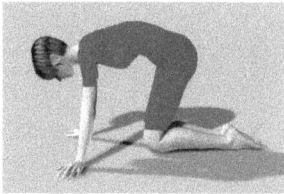

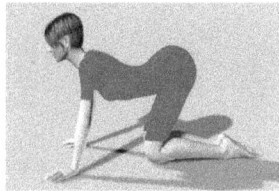

When ready to get up, sit up on hands and knees and perform a few cat stretches. Then sit on your heels stretching the hands in front in a dog stretch.

Rising into the downward dog, walk towards the hands and stand up with palms together.

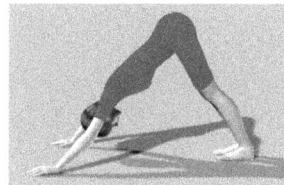

# Dhanvantri

Dhanvantri appeared in primordial times during the churning of the milky way by the Gods and Demi-Gods. Subsequently, he took birth as the son of the King of Kasi to formulate the healing system of Ayurveda for the benefit of humanity. He is the great Healer.

> *Enquire into and experience the teachings of the guru;*
> *The beginning and the end letters are ari Aum.*
> *To honor the Guru is to gain experience;*
> *The abode fo the Vashi is in the center of the body;*
> *Which is man and which is woman? Both becoming One;*
> *The still point is the gold.*
> *Vainly I do not state this wisdom;*
> *What I have revealed is the crown of knowledge.*
> > *Verse 8 Jnanam-12*

Posture 11

# Yogic Symbol Pose

## Benefits:

Energetic: stimulates the smooth rising of Kundalini energy; awakening of navel energy center

Mental / Spiritual: awakening to higher consciousness

Physical: expansion of chest capacity; strenghten nerves of hands

Therapeutic:
first variation: correction of lumbar lordosis; rheumatoid arthritis in the back
second variation: constipation
third variation: correction of contractures in shoulders, elbows and wrists

**Avoid this posture: heart disease; serious back conditions; after surgery; after giving birth**

**Affirmation used during holding phase: I am yours, receive me now**

Sanskrit Name: Yoga Mudrasanaa

Siddha: Dhanvantri

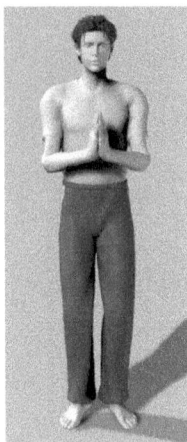

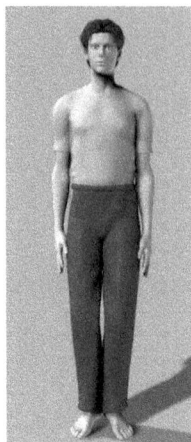

Stand erect with heels together and toes apart; the palms of the hands are placed together at the heart level. Lower the hands by the sides; shoulders and legs relaxed; eyes softly focused ahead.

First variation:

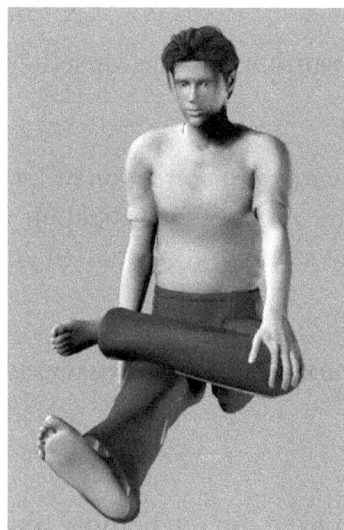

Sit down on the floor, crossing left foot in front of right. Place left foot on right thigh, gently stretch left knee up and down with left hand. Place right foot on left thigh, gently stretch right knee up and down with right hand.

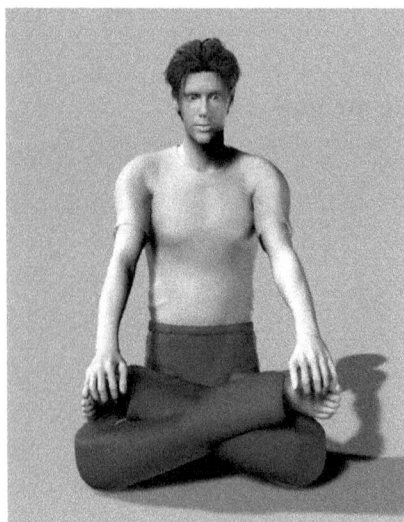

Place left leg on right thigh and right leg over left. This is the complementary lotus pose to the one used in posture #4.

If you are unable to place the right leg over the left, place it under in the half-lotus. If you have knee problems, use the simple cross-leg position.

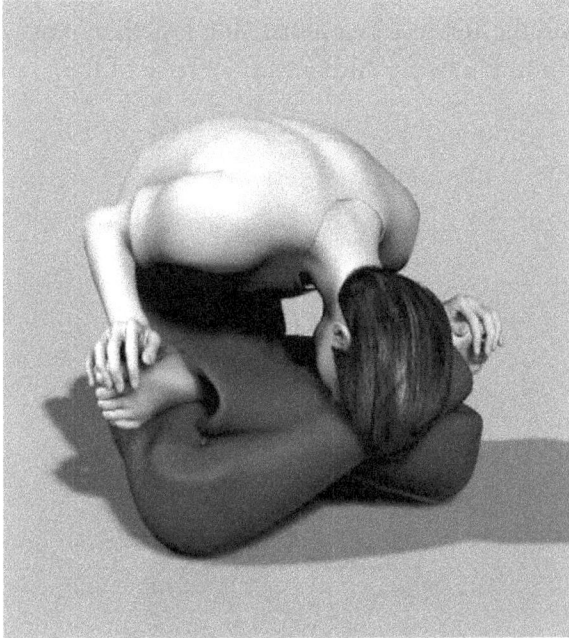

Grasp hold of the great toes. Bend forwards, keeping the seat on the floor. Elongate back, gently bend forwards several times. Bring forehead closer and closer to the floor; till touching, then nose, till touching, then chin. Hold the position for about 30 seconds. **Repeat the affirmation, "I am yours, receive me now."** Sit up and relax.

Second variation:
Join the two fists together at the level of the navel.

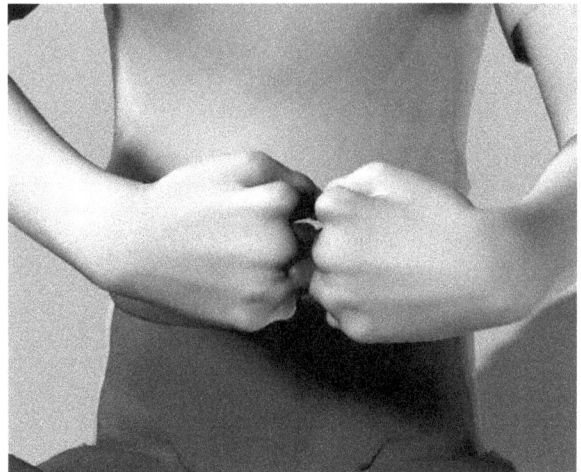

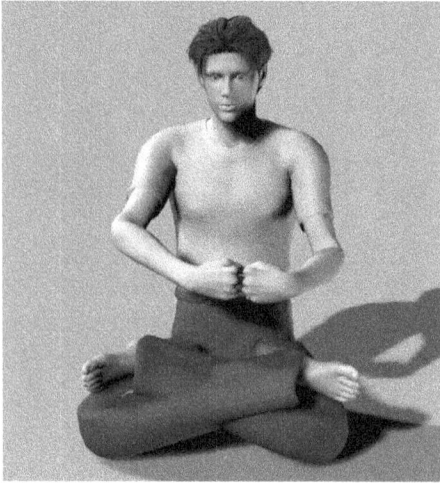

Roll the fist like gears meshing together, massaging the nerve endings at the base of the fingers.

Stop the movement; place fists together in the abdomen, bending forwards three to four times, pressing the fists into the lower abdomen.

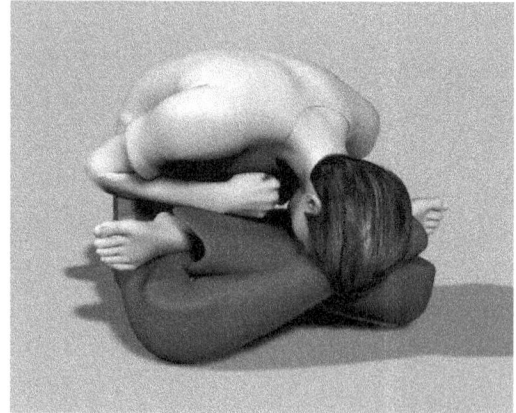

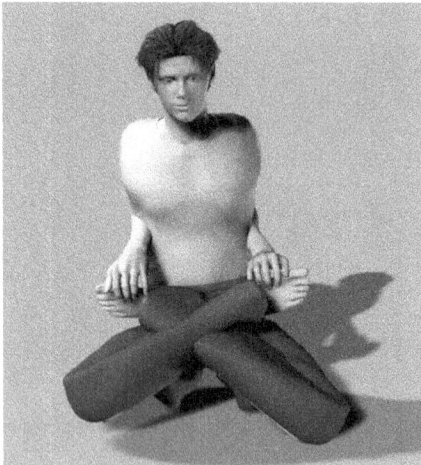

Third variation:
Cross arms behind back and reach towards opposite great toes, grabbing them if possible. Bend forwards three or four times. Lower arms and unwind legs. Straighten legs and flex them to relax for a minute or so. Stand up slowly with palms together.

# Konkanavar

Konkanavar was a seller of iron pots by trade and a householder with a large family. He would feed the yogis with cow's milk and they in turn fed him the milk of wisdom. In due time, when he was old, he became a renunciate and went into the forests to meditate. There, he came upon a village where a young man had died and there was great distress and mourning. He took pity on them and entered the dead body so that the parents and relatives would be happy. The villagers were very happy but puzzled by this extraordinary occurrence and soon discovered the true reason when they found the meditating body of Konkanavar. They promptly burnt the original body, forcing Konkanavar to remain in the youthful body. Later, the Siddha discovered the secrets of the herbs for longevity and achieved rejuventation of the body at will.

It is told that once, while he was meditating under a tree, a crane dropped excreta on him and when he opened his eyes in anger, the crane was burnt to ashes. The Siddha was hungry and went to a village to seek food. However, he was kept waiting for a long time by the woman of the house he had sought food from. When she finally came, he gave her a very angry look, whereupon the Divine Mother smiled and said, " Konkanavar, I'm not a crane, you know." The Siddha learnt a valuable lesson that day.

> *Remain firmly convinced that it is I*
> *Which is That; forget the rest.*
> *Gather the nectar and enjoy the bliss.*
> *My son, practice and enter samadhi.*
> *Announce that there is no evil or sin*
> *No fate, nor thought. Fly high.*
> *Do wander aimlessly like people who go nowhere.*
> *Remain steadfast in the Transcendence.*
> *Verse 2, Meyjnanam-13*

# Half Wheel Pose

## Benefits:

Energetic: activates the pituitary and pineal glands; awakens the crown chakra

Mental: improves memory

Physical: muscle toning

Therapeutic: kyphosis (hunch back); herniated disc or slipped disc

**Avoid this posture: heart disease or high blood pressure; arthritis of the neck**

**Affirmation used during holding phase: I am Awake and Ready! Energetic and Enthusiastic!**

Sanskrit Name: Ardha Chakrasana

Siddha: Konkanavar

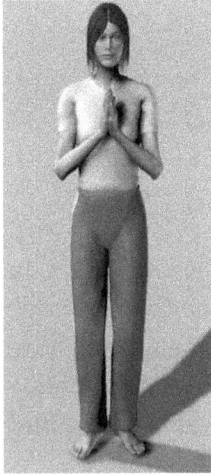

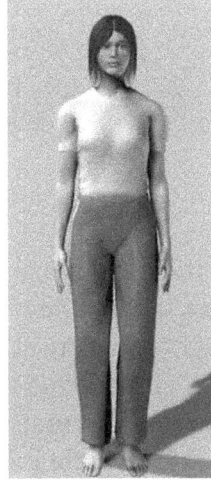

Stand erect with heels together and toes apart; the palms of the hands are placed together at the heart level. Lower the hands by the sides; shoulders and legs relaxed; eyes softly focused ahead.

Lie down on your back.

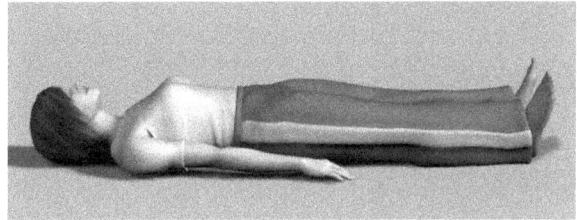

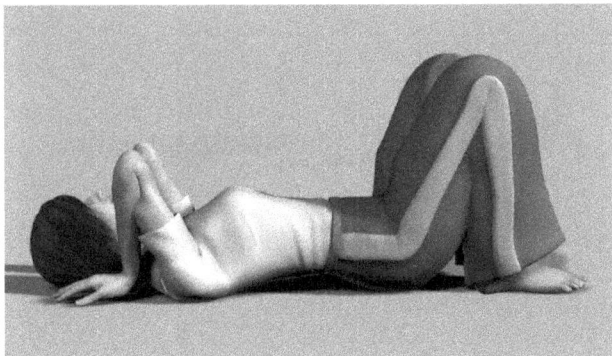

Place feet near your seat, shoulder width apart, knees up. Place hands near shoulders, elbows up.

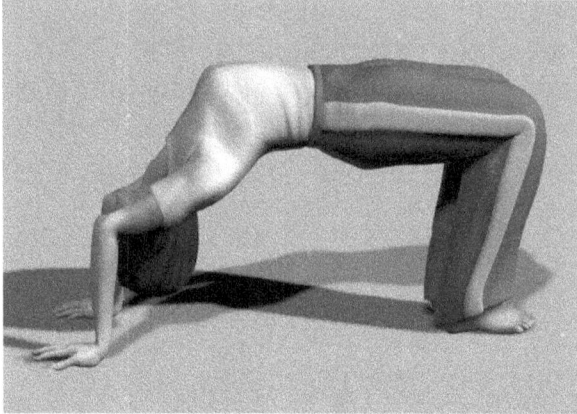

Raise trunk at least six inches. Allow the head to drop back, with the top on the floor. Distribute weight evenly between feet, hands and head. Breathe normally and hold for one minute. **Repeat the affirmation, "I am Awake and Ready! Energetic and Enthusiastic!"**

Press down with your hands to raise the head off the floor slightly and back to the starting position. Lower arms to side and lower legs to floor. Turn head and neck from side to side to release all tension. Relax for a minute or two.

Then raise your hands over your head; stretch. Sit up and touch your hands to your legs. Stand up with palms together at the heart level.

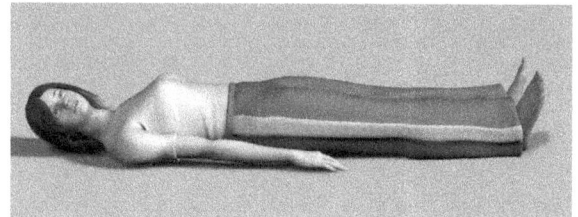

# Sundaranandar

Sundaranandar was a disciple of Sattamuni and lived in Cautagiri. Elsewhere, it is said that he was a disciple of Bhoganath. When Agastya came down from the Himalayas, he met him in Podigai hill, and was given the shivalinga worshipped by the Rishi.

He was such a great worshipper of the Shivanlinga that even Lord Shiva came down from Mt. Kailash to test him. Sundaranandar explained to the Lord who was masquerading as a Siddha, *"As I see the Lord everywhere, I see Him in this tiny idol also. Like the fire that exists in the stick concealed, the Lord resides here, in this idol and in me."*

> *The nectar of immortality cannot be attained by the lowly*
> *It is attained instantaneously by one who becomes Shiva-yogi*
> *The life essence is stopped from leaking out and moves up*
> *Transcendence will appear in the third-eye*
> *The body shines like the sun*
> *It is surprising like walking on the razor's edge!*
> *Mother Kundalini will come and impart the secret to you;*
> *Speak not the secrets; observe silence.*
> *Verse 8 Siva Yoga Jnanam-32*

Posture 13

# Sitting Crane Pose

Benefits:

Energetic: awakening of sacral chakra or 2nd energy center

Mental / Spiritual: harmony

Physical: toning of muscles and organs such as liver, kidneys, stomach and pancreas.

Therapeutic: reduce prostate in men;  lumbar lardosis

**Avoid this posture: kyphosis (hunchback)**

**Affirmation used: I live life with Joy!**

Sanskrit Name: Amarntha Kokkuasanaa

Siddha: Sundaranandar

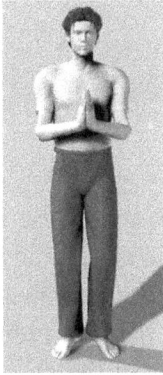

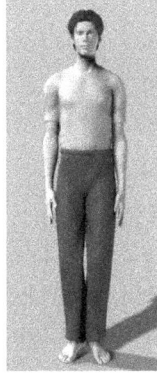

Stand erect with heels together and toes apart; the palms of the hands are placed together at the heart level. Lower the hands by the sides; shoulders and legs relaxed; eyes softly focused ahead.

Lie down on your back with arms by the side.

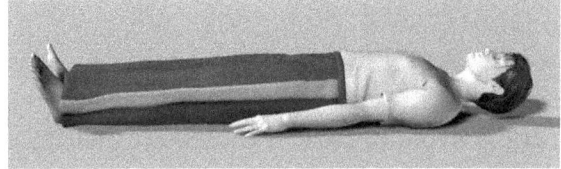

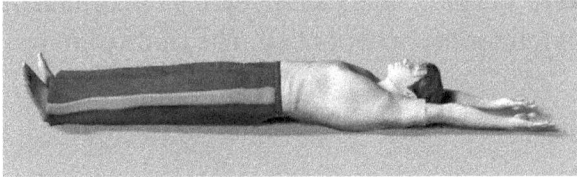

Stretch arms above head; sit up stretching hands towards the ceiling, elongating the back, the lower arms and head. and stretch hands above and beyond the feet in a gentle rocking motion. Keep the head down and keep legs flat on the floor.

Stop the motion, grab the big toes or ankles. Pull back forward and hold this position for one minute. Push heels forward, straighten legs, breathe in deeply to where you feel the tension and breathe it out. **Repeat the affirmation, "I live life with Joy!"** Lie back, stretching the arms above the head. lower arms to the sides and relax for a minute or two.

Then raise your hands over your head; stretch. Sit up and touch your hands to your toes. Stand up with palms together at the heart level.

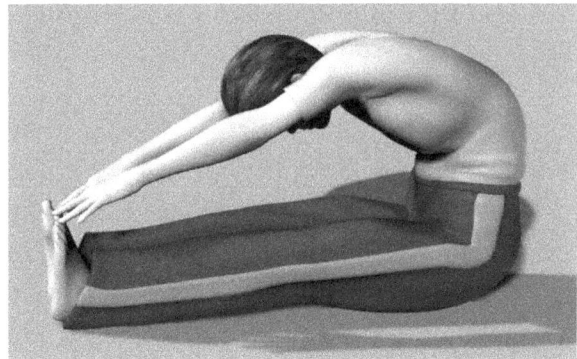

# Idai Kadar

It is said that this Siddha was shepherd who would herd his goats on a hillock and while they were grazing, he would stand with his eyes closed in samadhi under a tree, leaning on his herding staff. One day, one of the Nine Naths was passing through the sky and seeing this shepherd in superconsciousness, came down to investigate. When Idaikadar came out of his meditation, he paid reverence to the Mahasiddha and gave him goat's milk to drink. In turn, the Mahasiddha initiated the shepherd into wisdom and knowledge of the Divine.

One story has it that Idaikadar, being an expert astrologer, foretold the coming of famine and was prepared for it -- one of the ways was to train his goats to eat a drought-resistent plant which animals generally avoid because it caused drowsiness and had an unpleasant taste. While the others were suffering from the famine, the Siddha went on as usual - this puzzled the Planetary Gods who came down to investigate. He paid reverence to them by giving them the goat's milk, which being infused with the special plant, made the gods fall asleep. While they were sleeping, Idaikadar took the opportunity to re-arrange the planets and so the draught ended and rain fell for the benefit of all. The Gods were well-pleased by the Siddha's compassionate ruse.

> *Perform the worship of the Lord,*
> *This is the seed for Liberation*
> *The only way to reach perfection and total devotion*
> *Is by the Mother Power and Liberation, Oh, Shepherd!*
> *Verse 3 Poems*

Posture 14

# Locust (Grasshopper) Pose

## Benefits:

Energetic: stimulates the base chakra and sacral chakra or sexual center;

Mental / Spiritual: Increased awareness

Physical: strengthening muscles of buttocks, legs, and hips

Therapeutic: diabetes; infertility of women and impotence in men

**Avoid this posture: heart disease**

**Affirmation used during holding phase: Divine energy suffuses me from head to toe**

Sanskrit Name: Salabhasana

Siddha: Idai Kadar

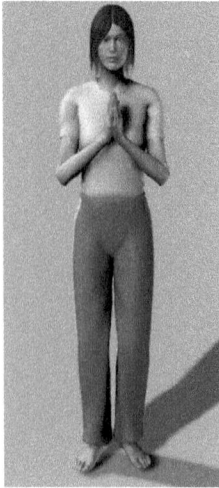

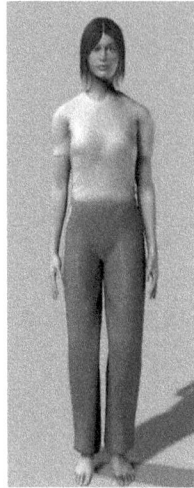

Stand erect with heels together and toes apart; the palms of the hands are placed together at the heart level. Lower the hands by the sides; shoulders and legs relaxed; eyes softly focused ahead.

Lie face down on the flow with hands by the side. Place the right hand a few inches away from the right hip.

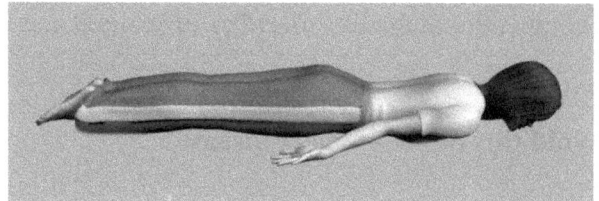

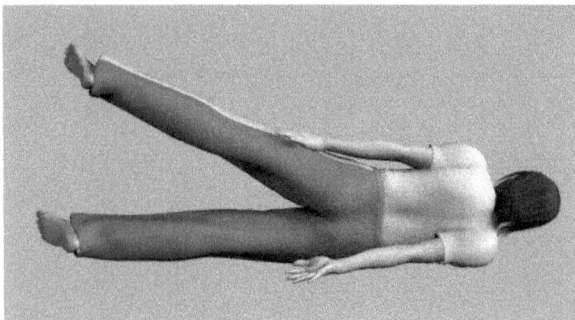

Raise the left leg from the hip and roll over onto the right side, keeping the left hand on the left thigh. Bend the right leg to support yourself and keep the side of the head on the floor; keep left leg straight and move it up and down in a scissors movement. Continue for ten repetitions. Stop the motion, roll back to the center and lower the leg.

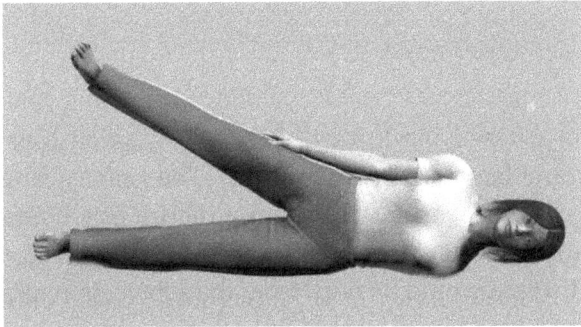

Place the left hand a few inches away from the left hip. Raise the right leg from the hip and roll over onto the left side, keeping the right hand on the right thigh. Bend the left leg to support yourself, keeping the side of the head on the floor. Keep the right leg straight as you move it up and down in a scissors movement.

Stop the motion and roll back to the center and lower the leg. **Repeat affirmation, "Divine energy suffuses me from head to toe."**

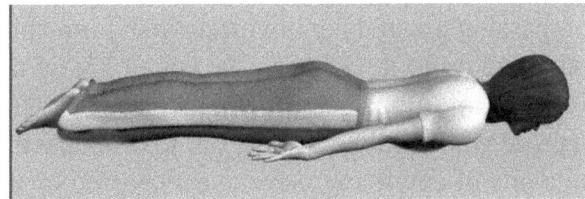

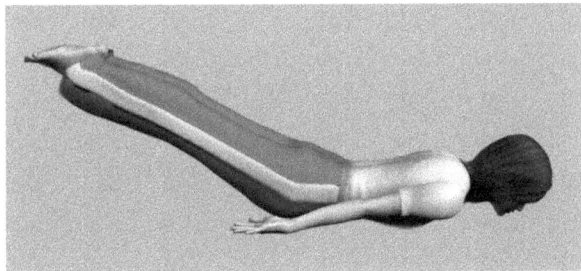

Raise both legs together from the hips, hold with arms relaxed by your sides and lower legs to relax. Repeat three times. Then relax and repeat affirmation, **"Divine energy suffuses me from head to toe."**

*Note that the affirmation in this posture is done during the relaxation phase rather than the holding phase because of its strenuousness.*

# Gorakshanath

Once Matsyendranath performed great austerities and pleased the Lord Shiva, who granted him a boon. The yogi repectfully asked for a disciple who would be greater than himself. The Lord of Yoga told Matsyendranath that he should ask for something else because it was impossible for any human being under the sun to be a greater yogi. However, Matsyendranath was persistent and finally the Lord agreed and gave him some ashes and told him that his disciple would be born from the ashes. In reality, Lord Shiva projected a part of Himself into the ashes and prepared to manifest in the human world.

During his travels, Matsyendranath came to a village and to the home of a virtuous but childless woman and asked her for food. She invited him into her home and fed him. He saw that she was sad and in compassion granted her unvoiced wish for a child by giving her the ashes and told her to put it in her water and drink it. However, he bound her by the condition that when the child was seven, she must give him up to become the yogi's disciple. Unfortunately, the woman had a sceptical and uncouth husband who would not allow her to drink the ashes but threw it out the window where it landed on a huge pile of cow-dung. Seven years passed by and Matsyendranath returned to the village to take his disciple. The sad woman confessed that the ashes had been discarded. Puzzled, since he could feel his disciple's presence, the great yogi called for the boy, who miraculously appeared from the cow-dung as a golden youth. He was called Gorakh. He was variously called Goraksha, Gorakhnath, or Gorakshanath, and became famous for his wisdom and miracles from Punjab to Bengal and from Nepal to Tamil Nadu. He is an immortal being guiding the spiritual evolution of humanity.

> *One who is established in his own luminosity*
> *Who has the luster of the nature of radiance*
> *Who delights in the world through play*
> *He can be called an Avadhut.*
> > *Verse 19, Pada 6, Siddha-Siddanta-Paddhati*

# Supine Pose of Firmness and Light

## Benefits:

Energetic: control of sexual energy; awakening of kundalini; increase of vital energy

Mental: stablity and brilliance

Physical: strengthens circulation and ovaries;

Therapeutic: infertility and impotence;

**Avoid this posture:**

**Affirmation used during holding phase: Divine light suffuses me from head to toe**

Sanskrit Name: Vajroli Mudrasana

Siddha: Gorakshanath

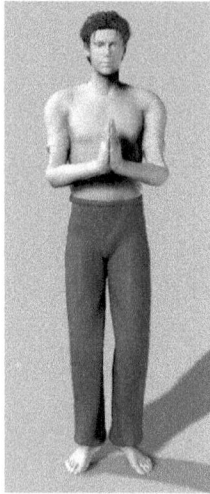

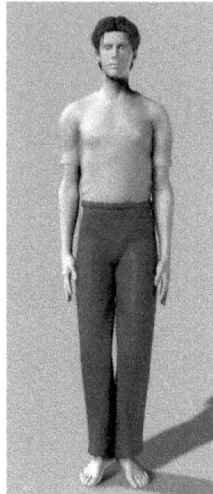

Stand erect with heels together and toes apart; the palms of the hands are placed together at the heart level. Lower the hands by the sides; shoulders and legs relaxed; eyes softly focused ahead.

Lie down on your back with hands by the side.

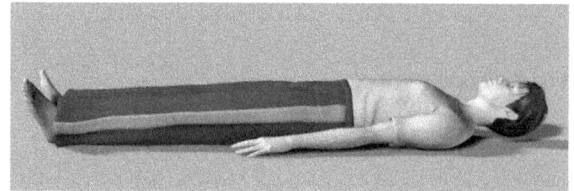

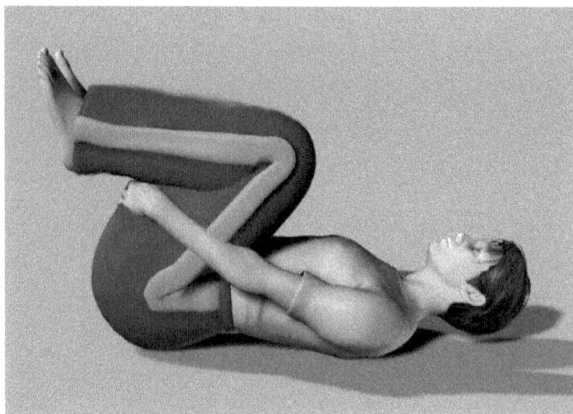

Raise legs off floor, keeping seat on floor. Clasp hands together behind knees.

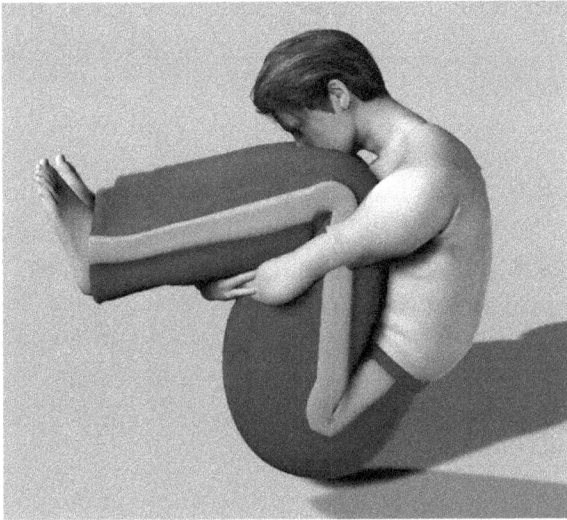

Sit up, balance on your seat with feet up. Move forehead close to the knees. Feel the energy from the base center along the spine to the third-eye. Hold for one minute. **Repeat affirmation, "Divine Light suffuses me from head to toe."**

Roll onto the back and bring the feet behind the head to a position where the knees touch the forehead.

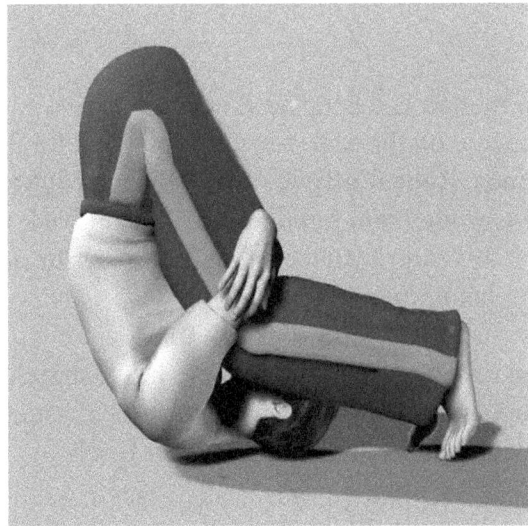

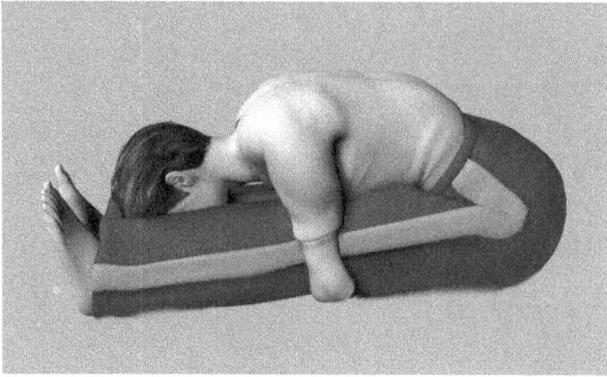

Roll forwards lowering the backs of the legs to the floor; slide heels on the floor and straighten legs, keeping head towards knees at all times. Repeat about seven times.

Stop motion and keep head near the knees, balancing on the seat. Keep this position for 30 seconds. **Repeat affirmation, "Divine Light suffuses me from head to toe."** Lower back to floor, lower arms to the sides; lower legs to floor and relax for a minute or two.

Then raise your hands over your head; stretch. Sit up and touch your hands to your legs. Stand up with palms together at the heart level.

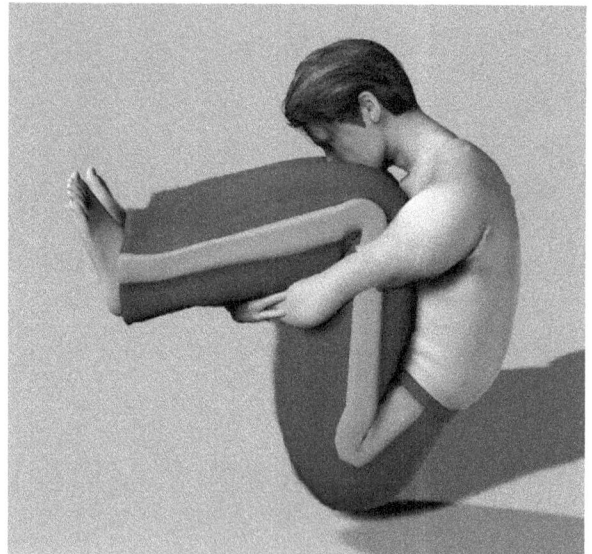

# Nandi Devar

A child called 'Sailadar', was born to the Rishi Silatatha who performed great austerities. From the very first, the child was devoted to Lord Shiva and practiced severe austerities. The Lord was pleased and asked the young man what he wished - Sailadar responded that he wished to always be with the Lord. This wish was granted, he was given the name Nandi which means joy and he became the head of Lord Shiva's retinue. Nandi was also given a cane to protect the good and destroy the evil.

Once Nandi was told that the Lord was angry with him because he was giving the high yogic teachings openly. He ran away and took the form of a bull, hiding in a secluded area. However, the Lord saw through the disguise and sweetly called him to come. Nandi came and in all humility knelt at the feet of the Lord and no-one dared to come between them. It is in the form of a bull that Nandi Devar is depicted in all Shiva temples and the tradition is that nobody should pass between Shiva and Nandi.

*After paying homage to the destroyer of obstacles*
*And after due reverence to the ever victorious Muruga,*
*One should revere Lord Shiva.*
*Recite namashivaya-krim-haum;*
*Hold this in its completeness;*
*Offer scented smoke, lights and eatables,*
*While praying to Sadashiva, who is glorious;*
*Who will grant all your wishes,*
*My son, all is in the Lord's power.*
　　　　　*Verse 3 Puja Vidhi-12*

# Kneeling Pose of Firmness

## Benefits:

Energetic: releasing energy from shoulders and back; stimulates kundalini at the base chakra

Mental / Spiritual: Attitude of Devotion

Physical: strengthen leg muscles

Therapeutic: prolapsed disc; sciatic nerve pain; improved digestion

**Avoid this posture: bad knees**

**Affirmation used during holding phase: I surrender myself to the Divine**

Sanskrit Name: Suptavajrasana

Siddha: Nandi Devar

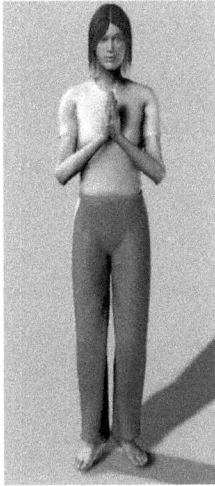

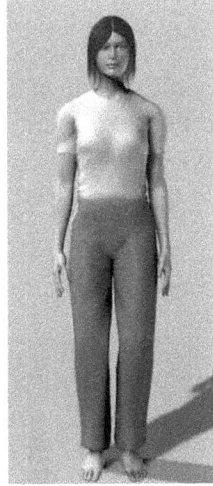

Stand erect with heels together and toes apart; the palms of the hands are placed together at the heart level. Lower the hands by the sides; shoulders and legs relaxed; eyes softly focused ahead.

Kneel down, knees together, feet together. Spread feet apart, keeping knees together. Sit between the feet.

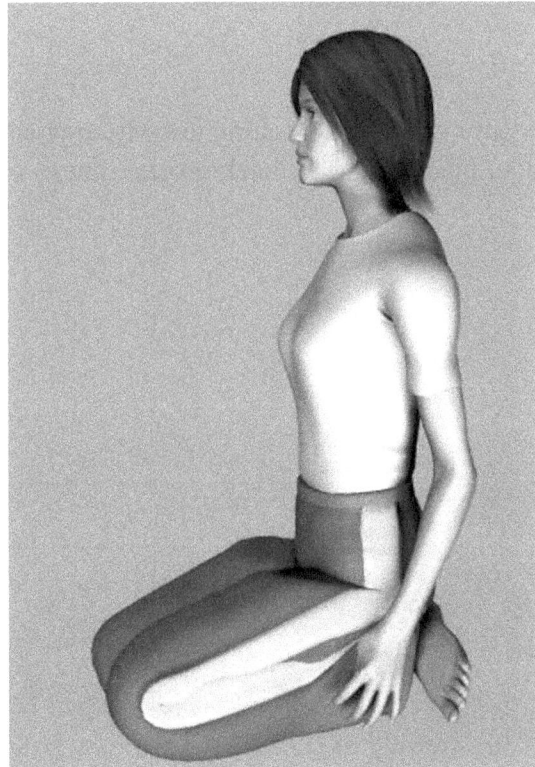

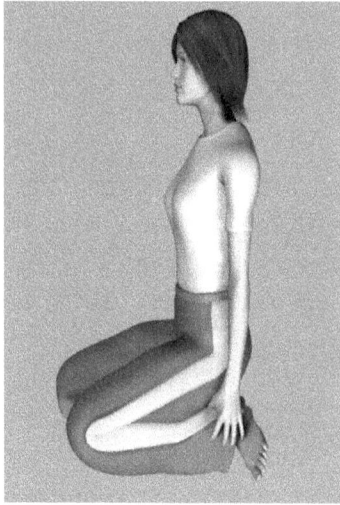

Hold onto the ankles; lift body up and lower it several times, bouncing the seat gently on the floor.

Cross arms over head reaching towards opposite shoulder blades; clap the back several times.

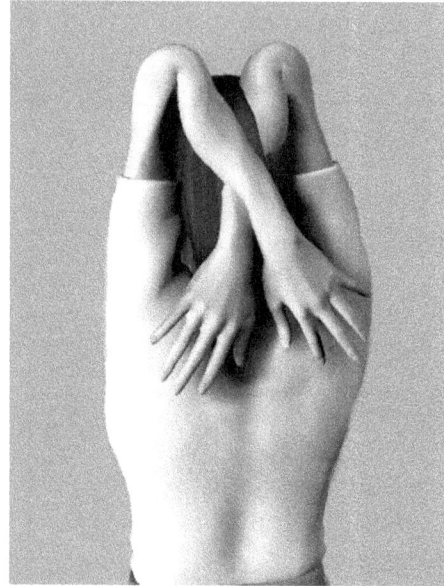

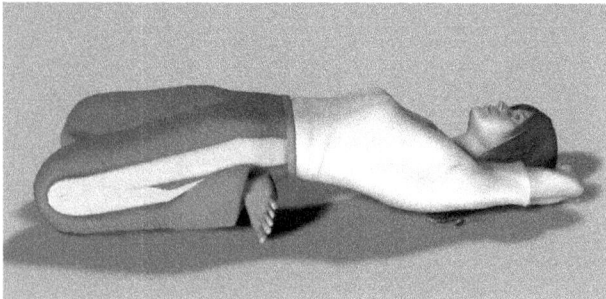

Lay back, lower head and shoulders to floor as far as possible. *Use hands to support yourself and lean back if you cannot reach the floor.* Hold this position and repeat the affirmation, **"I completely surrender myself to the Divine."** Cross arms behind the head and clap the back several times. Stop clapping, uncross arms. Use your hands to support yourself and sit up. Kneel up, bring feet together and stand up. Relax for a few moments.

# Agastya

So vast is this Being that it is not possible to estimate his time nor space. Agastya is one of the seven primordial sages who consitute seven stars. He is a son of the Mitra, the friendly light of Dawn.

When the demons hid in the seas from Indra, the Warrior King of the Gods, it was Agastya who drank the seas dry so that Indra could destroy them. Afterwards, the Rishi-Siddha filled the seas up by bringing the waters back out from his stomach.

During the time of Lord Shiva's wedding to Parvati, so many celestial beings went to the Himalayas, that the world was in danger of tipping over. Lord Shiva sent Agastya to the southern tip of the world to balance the weight. The Lord granted him the boon of witnessing the wedding festivities wherever he might be.

In the later time of King Rama, the Divine Incarnation of Lord Vishnu, it was Agastya who guided the warrior King to defeat Ravana, the demon King of Sri Lanka.

On another occassion, two demons who used to prey on innocent travellers met their match at the hands of the Rishi-Siddha. These two were brothers and one of them would take the form of a goat and the other would feed the goat meat to the unsuspecting guest. After the meal, the demon in the stomach would burst our killing the poor passer-by. When Agastya was invited for the meal, he smilingly accepted, but when the the second brother called the first to come out, there was no answer, as he had been digested. Agastya dispatched both demons that day.

*Grey hair, wrinkles of the skin, all diseases would vanish in the glorious state of samadhi;*
*The body complexion would be a glowing radiance;*
*The body would ever be in youthfulness of sixteen,*
*The life-force as Aum will become the internal body.*
    *verse from Poem on Samadhi*

# Triangle Pose

## Benefits:

Energetic: stimulates the whole nervous system and enhances energy flow through the energy channels

Mental / Spiritual: Postive Joy; optimism

Physical: strengthening of internal organs around abdomen

Therapeutic: correction of disorders of the vertebral column;

**Avoid this posture:**

**Affirmation used: Joyful energy flood every cell of my body**

Sanskrit Name: Trikonasana

Siddha: Agastya

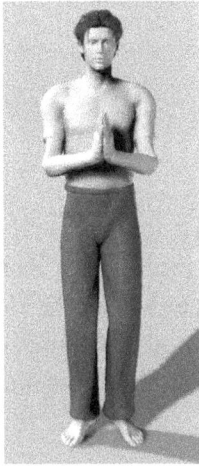

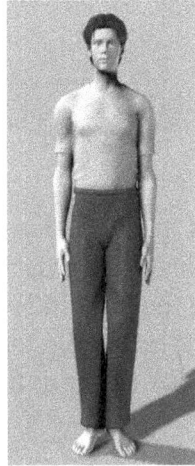

Stand erect with heels together and toes apart; the palms of the hands are placed together at the heart level. Lower the hands by the sides; shoulders and legs relaxed; eyes softly focused ahead.

Spread the feet apart and stretch the arms out to the sides. Look at the right index finger; lower the left index finger to the floor and mover it towards the left big toe; do not bend knees. Rotate and move the left index finger toward the right big toe. Rotate back, moving the left index finger back towards the left big toe. Stand up.

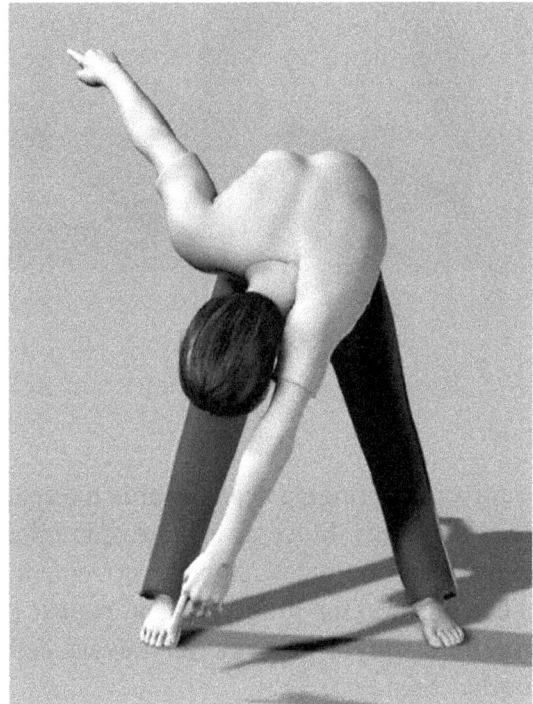

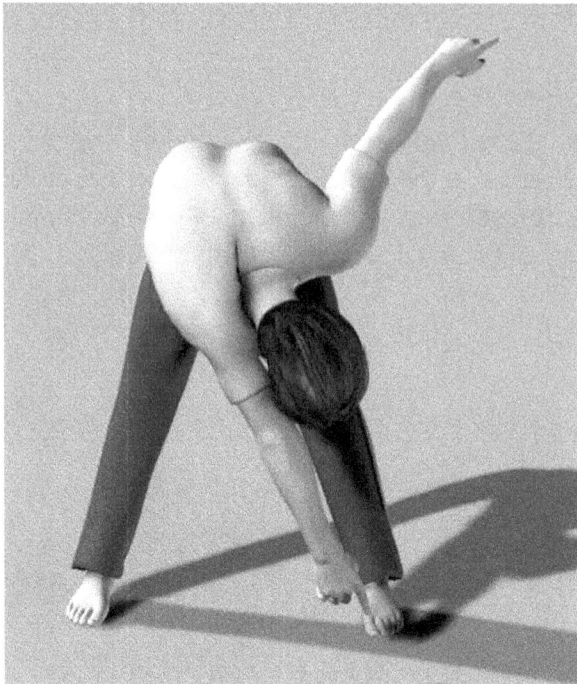

Look at the left index finger; lower the right index finger towards the right big toe. Rotate, moving the right index finger across the floor towards the left big toe. Rotate back moving the right index finger to the right big toe; stand up.

Bend forwards, bringing head towards the space between the knees. Move up and down in micro-movements several times. Stop the movement. Hold this position for 30 seconds and **repeat the affirmation, "Joyful Energy flood every cell of my body."** Stand up.

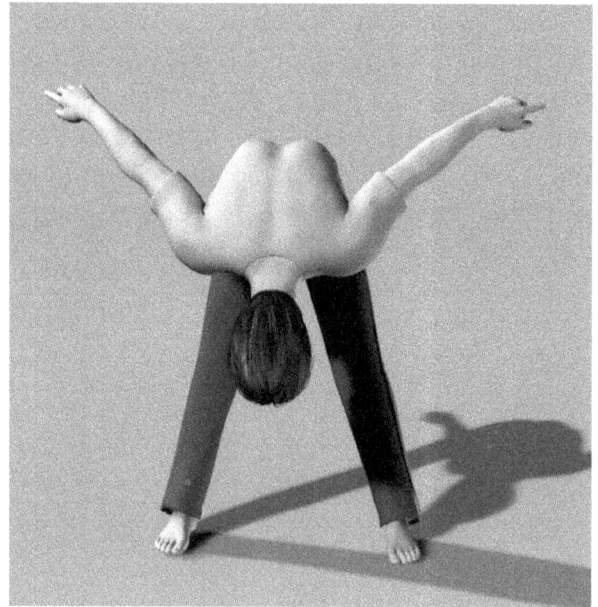

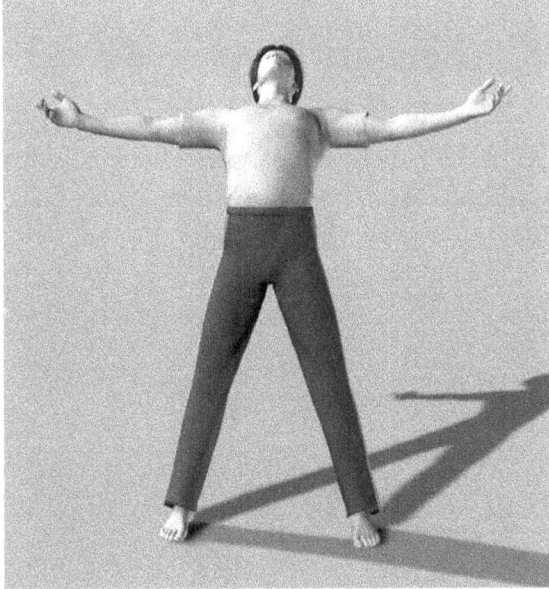

Bend backwards and hold for a few seconds. Straighten up to the verical position.

Keeping arms spread to the side, turn the trunk and shoulders to the right side. Bend forwards, bringing the head towards the right knee. Move back and fro in micro-movements. Stop the motion and stand up, still facing the right side.

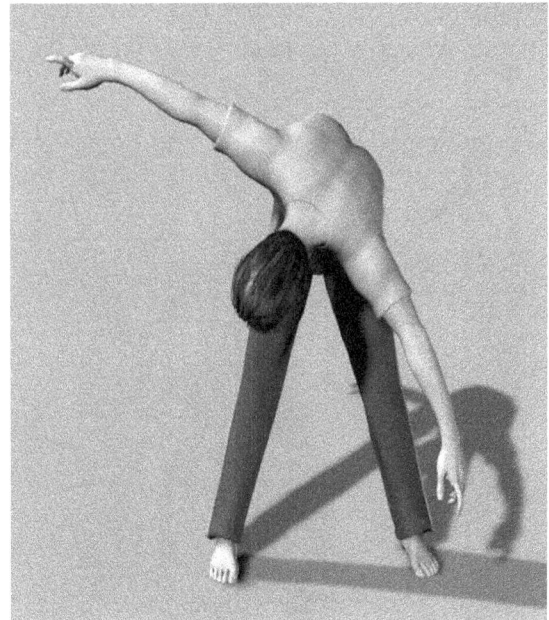

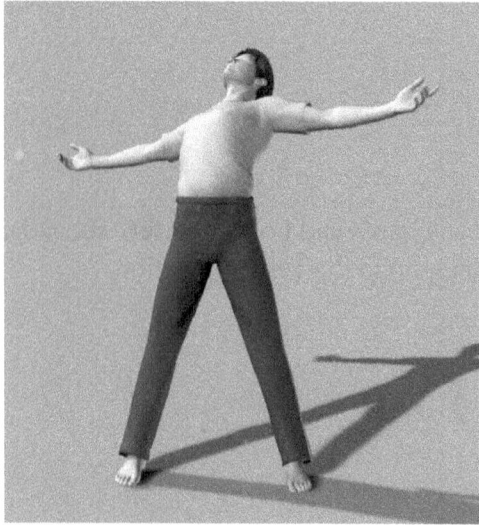

Bend backwards towards the left side; hold for a few seconds. Stand up straight and rotate back to the center.

Turn trunk and shoulders to the left side. Bend forwards, bringing head towards the left knee. Move up and down in micro-movements.

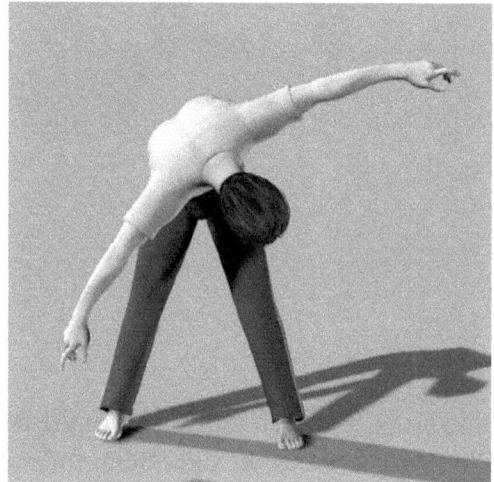

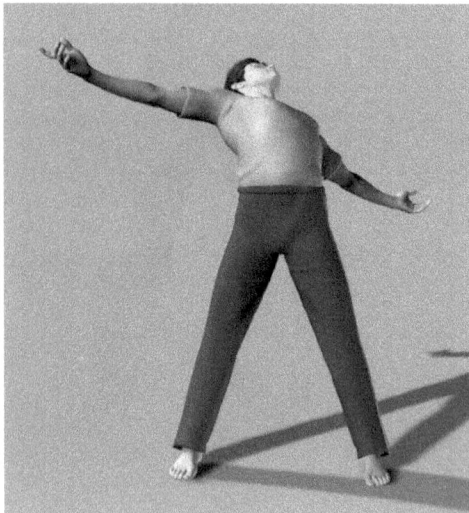

Stop movement and stand up, still facing the left side. Bend backwards towards the right side. Hold for a few seconds. Stand up straight, rotate back to the center. Lower arms to the sides, standing with heels together and toes apart. Relex, spreading the feet wider. Breathe deeply and slowly.

# Sattamuni

It is said that this Siddha was the son of a Sri Lankan prostitute who came to live in the Tamil region after his birth. Sattamuni became a householder but this ill-befitted him and when he had the opportunity, he ran away with a North Indian ascetic wearing a conch. Later he was initiated by Bhoganath.

Sattamuni angered some of the other Siddhas because he wrote in ordinary language rather in the coded language intended to prevent the uninitiated from learning the deeper knowledge. Some of his works were destroyed. Sattamuni defended himself by explaining that his poetry when learnt by the sincere acted as an initiation by itself!

On another occassion, the Siddha travelled to worship at a temple of Lord Aranganatha, but reached too late and the city gates were closed. He shouted the name of the Lord three times. Immediately, the gates opened and the temple bells started ringing and he was transported to the temple. The people came running and found him in meditation with the ceremonial clothing and jewellery from the image of the Lord. They accused him of stealing the jewels and took him to the King who saw that he was a holy person. Sattamuni once again shouted the Lord's name three times, "Aranga!, Aranga!, Aranga!" Again he was clothed in the ceremonial regalia. Everyone now understood that the Lord was trying to tell them that Sattamuni was one with the Lord.

> *It is known as the gracious Shiva-Yoga*
> *Also famous as Kundalini Mother.*
> *It is the vital breath, also the Yoga of firm seed.*
> *It is spoken of as Vashi Yoga, and understood as Hamsa.*
> *Good friend, Unite for realization of wisdom,*
> *Achieve then the imperishable body.*
> *Verse 4 Paripuranam-12*

# Complete Peace Relaxation

## Benefits:

Energetic: rejuvenation

Mental: peace; relief stress

Physical: relief physical stress, fatigue and tension.

Therapeutic: sciatica

**Avoid this posture:**


Affirmation used: *Om Shanti, Shanti, Shanti. Shalom, Sat Nam, Sadhu, Tao, Em, Aum, Spirit, Swami, Kami, Amin, Amen, Aumen, Selah, Hum, Aum.*


Sanskrit Name: Purna Shava Shanti asana

Siddha: Sattamuni

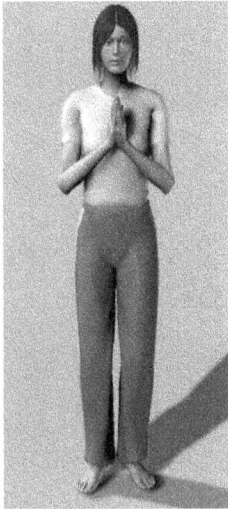

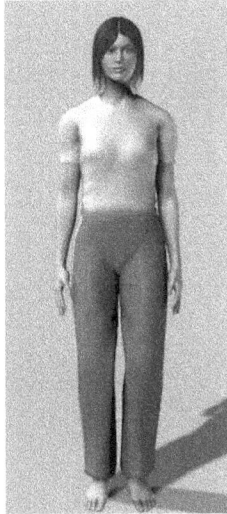

Stand erect with heels together and toes apart; the palms of the hands are placed together at the heart level. Lower the hands by the sides; shoulders and legs relaxed; eyes softly focused ahead.

Lie down on the back.

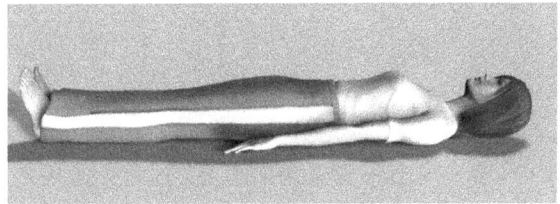

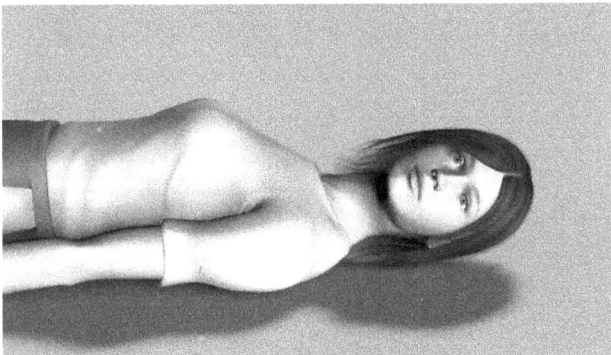

Turn the head and neck side to side to release tension in the neck; stop and relex.

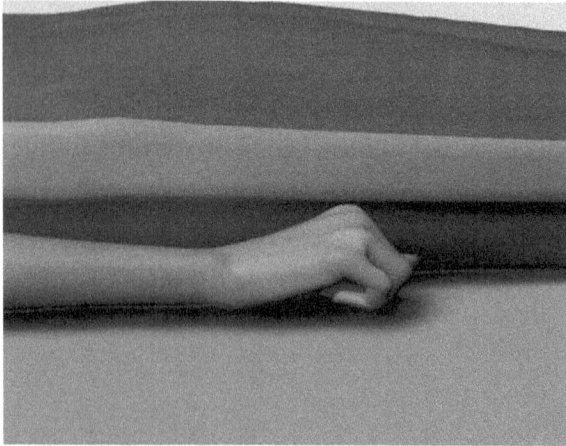

Grip thumb of the right hand with the fingers, forming a fist; squeeze hard, then relax.

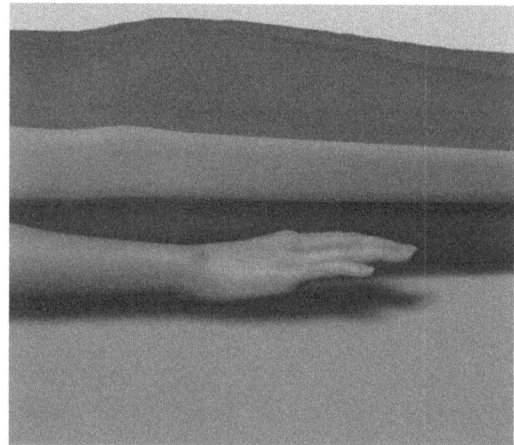

Raise the right forearm a few inches and let it fall.

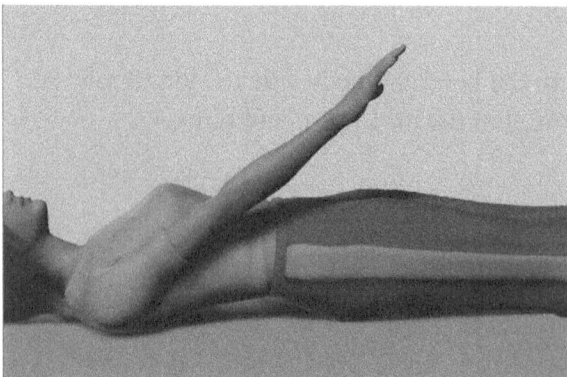

Raise the whole right arm from the shoulder, a few inches from the floor; let it fall.

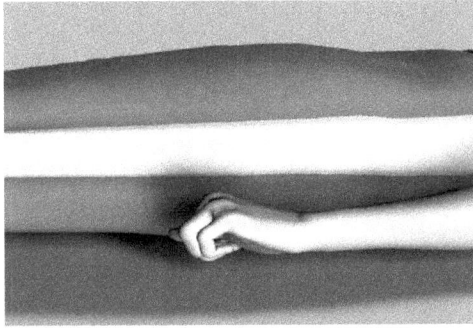

Grip thumb of the left hand with the fingers, forming a fist; squeeze hard, then relax.

Raise the left forearm a few inches and let it fall.

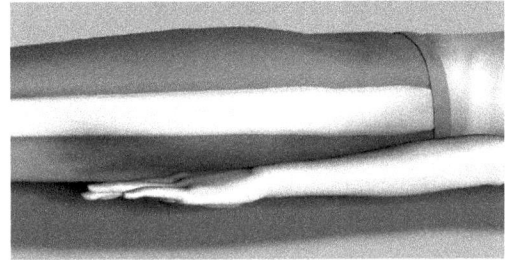

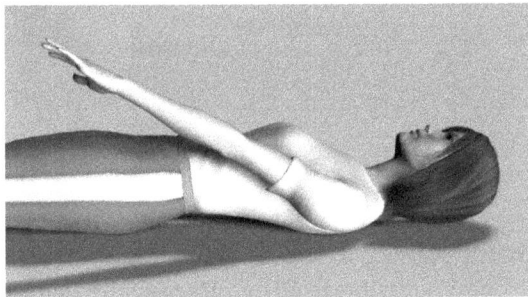

Raise the whole left arm from the shoulder, a few inches from the floor; let it fall.

Move toes of right foot back and forth, spread them apart; repeat with the left foot.

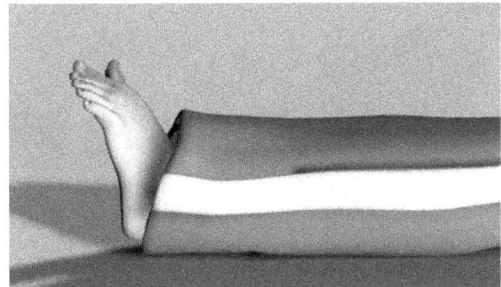

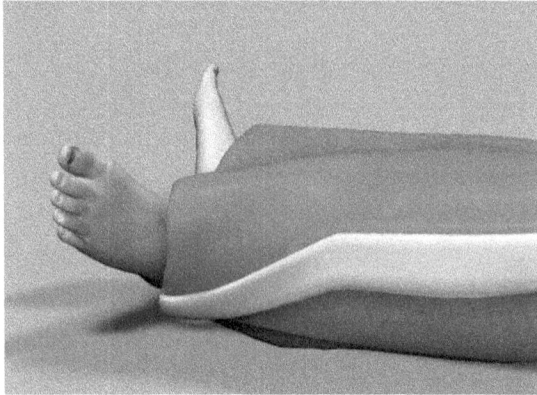

Rotate the feet side to side rolling on the heels.

Raise the right leg as whole a few inches; let it fall.

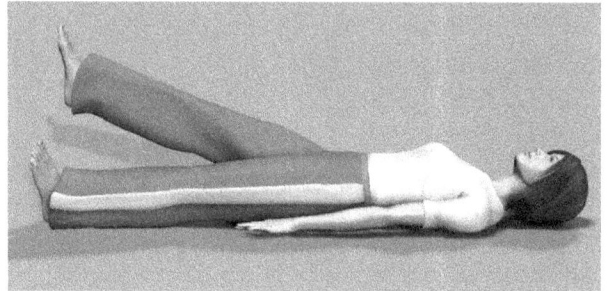

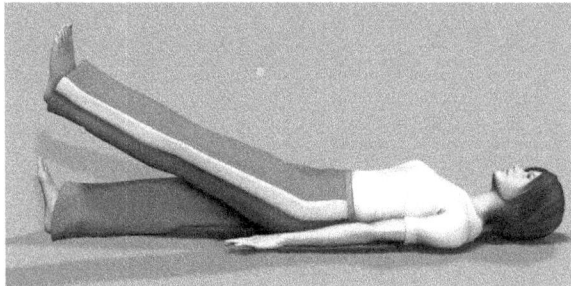

Raise the left leg as whole a few inches; let it fall. Relax your body fully. Repeat the Peace mantra to relax the mind also. Rest for a minute or two.

Then raise your hands over your head; stretch. Sit up and touch your hands to your legs. Stand up with palms together at the heart level.

# Pranayama
## Practice of Life-Force Control and Expansion throught the Breath

*Once the physical body has been exercised, we should begin the practice of Pranayama. This is the expansion and control of the life-force energy prana and exercises the energy body. The medium for controlling the prana is through the breath, but one should never lose sight of the fact that it is the prana carried by the breath that is the object of the practice.*

*note: for a more thorough study of the profound science of breath, please refer to the author's work published by Alight Publications,* **Breathe Like Your Life Depends On It**.

# Warm-up

Stand with your feet together and your arms by your sides. Slowly take a long, deep inhalation as you slowly raise your arms above your head, stretch right up onto your toes and pull your shoulders back as you stretch your arms up above your head. Then as you exhale, slowly lower your arms back down to your sides. Repeat five times.

Stand with the feet hip-width apart and inhale as you raise your arms above your head. Keep your arms straight, but with your hands and wrist relaxed. Exhale as you rotate your arms forward in a wide circle. Inhale as you raise your hands and exhale as you lower them. Practice the forward motion of the arms for five rounds then change direction and rotate them back in a reverse motion.

# Cleansing Breath

This breath is very beneficial for ventilating and cleansing the lungs. It stimulates the cells and gives a good tone to the respiratory organs. It also eliminates carbon dioxide from the system.

Caution: This exercise should not be practiced by those with heart problems or with abnormal blood pressure.

1. *Standing position:*
   Stand with your feet shoulder width apart, arms relaxed by your sides. Take a complete breath, and raise your hands over your head. Then with your lips puckered, exhale the breath out powerfully making a 'whoosh' sound, as you slowly bend at the knees to bring your hands between your knees and towards the floor. Slowly inhale through your nostrils as you rise up and bring the hands overhead again. Perform this three times.

2. *Sitting position:*
   Sit comfortably cross-legged on the floor with spine straight and body relaxed. Place your hands on your knees. Inhale a complete breath. Then pucker your lips and exhale vigorously through them in a series of short, sharp exhalations as you slowly lower your trunk and forehead as close to the floor as possible. Then slowly raise your head and trunk back up while slowly breathing in through the nostrils. Perform this three times.

3. *Alternate nostril cleansing:*
    Sit in a comfortable posture with your spine straight and body relaxed.

    Slowly inhale through both nostrils, then pucker your lips and exhale all the air from your lungs with a series of dynamic exhalations, like a bellows action.

    Keeping the breath out, close the right nostril with your right thumb and inhale through the left nostril.

    Then close your left nostril with the little and ring fingers of your right hand and exhale through your right nostril, with a series of short, sharp exhalation.

    Continue with inhaling through the right nostril, and exhaling through the left. Start the cycle again with inhaling through both nostrils.

    Practice three rounds.

    This is especially beneficial for those suffering from sinus congestion.


# Sukha Pranayama or Simple Calming Breath

This is an excellent breathing technique for reducing stress and producing a calm mind.

    Sit comfortably, keeping a smiling face, and relaxed body. Inhale slowly, but without strain from both nostrils, and then exhale slowly through both nostrils.

    Feel your body being energized by the breath. Mentally count the duration of the inhalation and try to make the exhalation to be of the same number of counts.

    It takes practice to count the duration of your breath, but after a little while, it will be second nature. The key at the beginning is to count consistently, and not vary the speed of the count.

Continue for twelve rounds. After the inhalation or the exhalation, if there is a natural pause, don't force the breath, and wait for the continuation. Your respiratory system will take care of your breathing.

It is generally recommended that you begin with a count of six, moving to twelve, after several weeks of practice.


# Nadi shuddhi: Alternate Nostril Breathing

*Nadi shuddhi* is the most important *pranayama* for purifying the *nadis* or energy channels in your energy body and for strengthening the nerves of the physical body. It purifies the blood and the brain cells, and also maintains equilibrium in the catabolic and anabolic processes in the body.

By making the breath flow in each nostril in a balanced way, the *pranic* flow in the *left* and *right nadis* become balanced. Under these balanced conditions, *prana* will flow into the *sushumna* or central channel, awakening the *Kundalini, or* dormant potential energy in your body.

Sit comfortably on the floor with legs crossed and with the head, neck and spine in a straight line. Keep a smile on your face and the body relaxed.

Place your left hand on your left knee, relaxed.

First, exhale through both nostrils, and then close your right nostril with your thumb and inhale slowly and deeply through your left nostril. Mentally count the duration of the inhalation. Close your left nostril with your ring and little fingers, release your thumb and exhale through your right nostril, making the exhalaling twice as long as the inhalation. Continue by inhaling through your right nostril, then close it with your thumb and exhaling through your left nostril.

Begin with a minimum inhalation count of six and exahalation count of twelve. After a week of practice, move to inhalation of eight and exahalation of sixteen.

This completes one round. Practice at least six rounds.

# Practice of Meditation

## Control of the mind and expansion into higher consciousness

*Once the life-force energy is under control and utilized for spiritual evolution, then it is time to put the mind under control and to expand beyond the limited mind into higher consciousness which can bring about a peace of mind, calmness and relief from stress. Eventually bliss and superconsciousness can be within one's experiential locus. There are hundreds of meditations techniques. The following one is well-suited as a progression from the 18 Postures and the Pranayama in the previous sections.*

# Hamsa Meditation

## Sitting Position:

Sit relaxed on the floor with crossed-legs; or on the edge of a chair; or even leaning back on a wall. One should not lay down on the floor as it is easily transitioned into a sleep state. The back should be straight without undue tension. The hands can be clasped and on the thighs or with the back of the right hand on top of the left palm. Eyes are closed.

## Technique:

Watch the breath. Do not attempt to force or control the breathing - let the body do its autonomous work. During this time, you may focus on the breath entering and leaving your nostrils. If the breath stops for any length of time, just wait and enjoy the calmness between breaths. Watch the breath for at least 5 minutes.

Next, as the breath enters, mentally repeat the syllable "SA" and as the breath is exhaled, repeat the syllable "HAM" (pronounced as in word hum.) Perform this watchful breath with the mystic sounds for 5 minutes.

Now, move your awareness to the third-eye center which is located inside your brain in the hollow space known as the third ventricle. This can be sensed by simultaneously moving your awareness down from the middle of the top of your head and moving inwards from the middle of the eyebrows - it is at the intersect of these two lines. Keep your attention here while you continue the repetition of the "SA" with inhalation and "HAM" with exhalation for another 5 minutes.

Expand your awareness to the space beyond the top of your head and around your body. Reverse the sounds for the breath -- inhale with "HAM" and exhale with "SA" for as long as you have the time. As you practice this, feel yourself expanding further and further and higher and higher into higher consciousness. Conclude by sensing your body and taking a few deep breaths before getting up.

OM Shanti -- Peace, Peace and everlasting Peace!

*Note: "SA" denotes the Divine and "HAM" denotes the I-Self. Hamsa is the symbol of the Soul. In the beginning, we aspire to the Divine with "That (Divine) I am" while in the ultimate, we realise, "I am That (Divine)"*

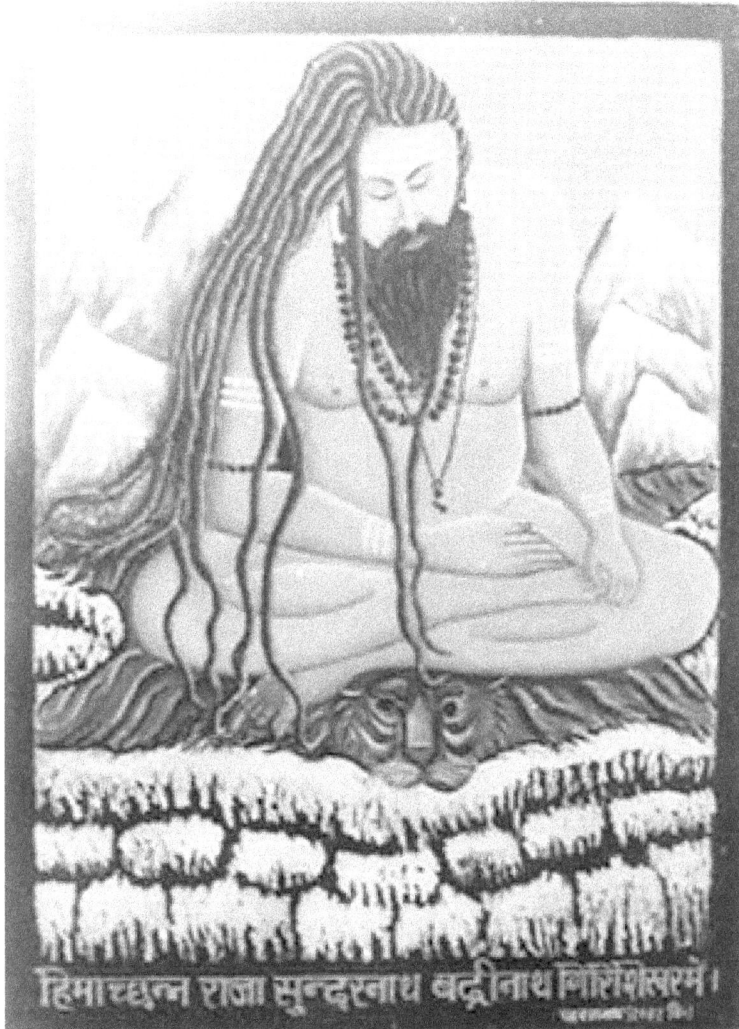

The great Siddha Sundarnath

# More Books by Rudra Shivananda

Chakra self-Healing by the Power of Om
Breathe like your Life depends on It
Surya Yoga (out of print)
The Yoga of Purification and Transformation
In Light of Kriya Yoga

## About the Author

*Rudra Shivananda* is dedicated to the service of humanity through the furthering of human awareness and spiritual evolution. He teaches that the only lasting way to bring happiness into one's life is by a consistent practice of awareness and transformation.

*Rudra Shivananda* is committed to spreading the message of the immortal Being called *Babaji*. He teaches the message of World and Individual Peace through the practice of *Kriya Yoga*. A student and teacher of Yoga for more than 30 years, he is initiated by his Master Yogiraj Gurunath Siddhanath as an *Acharya* or Spiritual Preceptor in Kriya Yoga and the Indian *Nath* Tradition, closely associated with the *Siddha* tradition. He is also experienced as a *Shakti* Healer and Astrologer with expertise in the healing and spiritual uses of mantras, gemstones and essential oils. He lives and works in the San Francisco Bay area, and has given initiations and workshops in USA, Ireland, India, England Spain, Russia, Brazil, Japan and Australia, Singapore, Malaysia and Hong Kong.

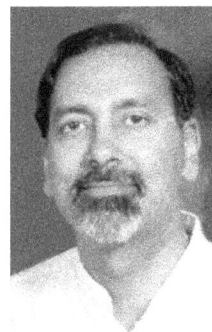

www.ingramcontent.com/pod-product-compliance
Lightning Source LLC
Chambersburg PA
CBHW081158270326
41930CB00014B/3200